AF874115

CHALLENGING SCENARIOS IN CLINICAL MEDICINE

First published 2025

Copyright © Dr Omar Hassouna 2025

The right of Dr Omar Hassouna to be identified as the author of this work has been asserted in accordance with the Copyright, Designs & Patents Act 1988.

All rights reserved. No part of this book may be reproduced, stored in a retrieval system, or transmitted in any form or by any means, digital, electronic, electrostatic, magnetic tape, mechanical, photocopying, recording or otherwise, without the written permission of the copyright holder.

The content of this book is for informational purposes only and is not intended to diagnose, treat, cure, or prevent any condition or disease. This book is not intended as a substitute for consultation with a licensed practitioner. Readers should consult with a qualified healthcare professional for any medical concerns or before making any decisions related to their health. The use of this book implies your acceptance of this disclaimer. The author and publisher are not liable for any damages or injuries resulting from the use of this book.

Published under licence by Brown Dog Books and
The Self-Publishing Partnership Ltd, 10b Greenway Farm, Bath Rd,
Wick, nr. Bath BS30 5RL, UK

www.selfpublishingpartnership.co.uk

ISBN printed book: 978-1-83952-965-8
ISBN e-book: 978-1-83952-966-5

Cover design by Kevin Rylands
Internal design by Andrew Easton

Printed and bound in the UK

This book is printed on FSC® certified paper

FSC
www.fsc.org
MIX
Paper | Supporting responsible forestry
FSC® C013604

CHALLENGING SCENARIOS IN CLINICAL MEDICINE

A CASE-BASED APPROACH TO CLINICAL REASONING

DR OMAR HASSOUNA

BROWN DOG BOOKS

Introduction

This book is a collection of real-life cases that I encountered during my career across various medical settings, including out-of-hours services, acute emergency centres, hospital wards and general practice. These cases vary significantly in type and context, presenting unique challenges for clinicians.

For instance, you might face a critical issue at midnight when no hospital beds are available, leaving you to decide the best course of action independently. Alternatively, you may encounter patients discharged prematurely, only to return repeatedly to emergency services or surgeries, still highly unwell. Such situations often place GPs in dilemmas, particularly when patients are left without adequate care, creating risks for their safety and potential litigation concerns.

In this book, I provide clear, actionable guidance on how to navigate these scenarios effectively and safely. By addressing these real-world challenges, the book equips GPs, junior doctors, and emergency clinicians with the tools and confidence to manage complex cases while ensuring patient safety and minimising legal risk.

Professional Profile

Name: Dr Omar J Hassouna

Title: General Practitioner, Author, Former Chair of Local GPs

With nearly five decades of experience working in the National Health Service (NHS), have dedicated my career to mastering a wide spectrum of medical specialties and contributing to healthcare in diverse ways. My journey began in 1976 in London, where completed my clinical attachment. From there, embarked on a purposeful path across various specialties, accumulating invaluable insights and expertise.

DIVERSE MEDICAL EXPERIENCE.

My early career included roles in paediatrics, geriatric acute medicine in Wales, and psychiatry, where I gained a deep understanding of mental health conditions such as anxiety and psychosis. These experiences shaped my holistic approach to patient care. As a medical registrar, further gained experiences in diabetes, haematology, respiratory medicine, cardiology, and gastroenterology, immersing myself in the complexities of these fields. I also briefly explored gynaecology and obstetrics, further broadening my scope of knowledge.

TRANSITION TO GENERAL PRACTICE

In 1983, I transitioned to general practice, joining a training practice before becoming a partner in 1984. This shift required significant adaptation as I expanded my focus to include the wide array of issues encountered in general practice. Established and managed several general practice clinics, including antenatal, postnatal, hypertension, diabetes, respiratory (COPD and asthma), thyroid and gout clinics. These services allowed us to address community health needs comprehensively.

To serve travellers, I established a WHO-Recognised Travel Clinic, providing guidance on travel risks, administering necessary vaccinations such as yellow fever and issuing certificates. This clinic was instrumental in supporting both our local community and patients from the practice.

LEADERSHIP AND ADMINISTRATIVE CONTRIBUTIONS

From 2007 to 2010, I served as Chair for the local GPs. In this role, I attended monthly Primary Care Trust (PCT) meetings and chaired a variety of GP meetings. This leadership position deepened my understanding of the administrative processes linking grassroots practices to the government's healthcare agenda. By fostering collaboration between GPs and PCT staff, I improved communication and facilitated smoother implementation of healthcare policies.

OUT-OF-HOURS AND URGENT CARE WORK

I worked extensively in out-of-hours (OOH) services during the 1980s and 1990s. Unlike today's systems, this work involved being on the road without the convenience of mobile phones and often in challenging weather conditions. These experiences taught me resilience, adaptability, and problem-solving skills. Later, with the advent of Urgent Care Centres after 2000, the nature of urgent care shifted, presenting new challenges and opportunities to serve patients effectively.

FORENSIC AND SOCIAL MEDICINE

In addition to general practice, I served as a police surgeon, working closely with law enforcement on cases involving drug abuse, assaults, sexual offences and deaths. This role provided a unique perspective on societal challenges and required collaboration with courts and police stations. I also worked with social services, assessing patients for disability and mobility allowances. Visiting patients in their homes offered deeper insights into the social determinants of health, further enriching my practice.

LIFELONG LEARNING AND SPECIALISATION

Committed to continuous improvement, I earned diplomas in Dermatology (Cardiff University) and Diabetes Care (Warwick University). These qualifications enhanced my ability to manage specialised clinics and address patient needs effectively.

REFLECTIONS ON THE NHS

Over the years, I have witnessed significant changes in the NHS, particularly since 2005. The system has struggled to cope due to factors such as the emigration of skilled doctors, population growth, aging demographics, inadequate resources and administrative inefficiencies. Staff morale has declined, and patients' needs have become increasingly complex. These challenges inspired me to contribute solutions through my writing.

AUTHORSHIP AND THOUGHT LEADERSHIP

Drawing on decades of experience, I am in the process of authoring two books:

1. *Challenging Scenarios in Medicine*: A practical guide for GPs and junior doctors, addressing real-life cases in general practice, A&E, hospital wards, and on the road. The book emphasises safe, effective medicine and offers strategies for managing complex challenges.
2. *How to Make Diagnosis Easier:* This book provides a structured framework for reaching diagnoses quickly and effectively. By focusing on common conditions and practical cases, it aims to save time, reduce costs and ensure patient safety.

Both books address modern healthcare challenges, such as premature discharges, resource shortages, and the rising demand for mental health services. They aim to empower healthcare professionals with practical tools to navigate today's medical landscape.

VISION FOR THE FUTURE

My career reflects a commitment to improving patient care, fostering collaboration and mentoring future generations of healthcare professionals. Through my writing and ongoing contributions, I aim to support colleagues in addressing the complexities of modern medicine and shaping a brighter future for healthcare.

Case study 1

INTRODUCTION

This patient was a twenty-two-year-old male Caucasian, in his final year of studying Law at university. He came from the north of England. He was a social drinker but never smoked. He was living in a ground floor flat with his girlfriend (a medical student in her fourth year).

Around 4 am on a very cold winter's night in 1986, the controller from the out-of-hours central office asked me to see a twenty-two-year-old male in a city suburb approximately six miles away from the city centre.

SYMPTOMS

The patient was lying on the sofa, in reasonable comfort. He stated that the previous night he had been out with his girlfriend to a Greek restaurant. They enjoyed their meal. Approximately 2am, he woke up with severe abdominal pain, in the central part, no radiation, with persistent vomiting. The pain was unbearable. He used hot water bottles to ease the pain slightly. He had no diarrhoea, no blood in the vomit, no urinary symptoms, or skin rash.

His girlfriend was concerned, as she was not affected and being a medical student, she decided to call the out-of-hours service.

PAST MEDICAL HISTORY

Regarding his previous medical history, he did not have any illnesses, was not allergic to known substances and was not on any regular medication.

EXAMINATION

The patient was a pleasant man and looked reasonably comfortable. He was not anaemic clinically, had no jaundice, no obvious skin rash or photophobia; he was hydrated. Temperature, 37.2, p 88/SR, neck, no stiffness, BP 120/65, heart unremarkable, chest clear. Abdominal examination, no lumps or distention, soft with minimal discomfort centrally, no rebound tenderness or rigidity. Spleen and liver not palpable clinically.

At end of the of examination, I had a long discussion with both and explained that now there were no signs to indicate any serious medical problems. I pointed out that there were no signs to indicate acute appendicitis. The pain could possibly relate to the meal they had the previous night, even though the girlfriend did not show any symptoms. It could also be a viral infection.

Both were happy with my explanation.

Advised the patient to keep himself hydrated, with sufficient liquid intake, and see how he got on. He should go and see his GP or contact our service should he need to do so.

SUBSEQUENT DEVELOPMENTS

A month later, I received a written complaint. The reason given was that failed to diagnose appendicitis. Apparently after four days of initial consultation, the patient had called his GP, and he was referred to the local hospital for possible acute appendicitis. He was operated upon. The surgeon who performed the operation said to him, "You were very lucky to arrive at the right time; your appendix was just about to burst, your life was saved. I cannot comment on the consultation with the previous doctor consultation."

I must admit, was surprised to receive this complaint,

believe I did everything in this case to a reasonable, accepted and professional standard. I believe, two issues generated this complaint:

Firstly, lack of understanding (patient perspective) about how illnesses may present themselves. Initially there may be vague non-specific abdominal pain. But then later, the picture may get clearer, though it is still hard to get an accurate diagnosis of acute appendicitis, as in a substantial number of appendectomy operations, the appendix proves to be normal.

Secondly, the negative comment made by the operating surgeon was crucial in lodging a formal complaint.

DIAGNOSTIC COMPLEXITY

Presentation of acute appendicitis can be challenging. It depends on several factors: one is the anatomical location of the appendix:

In the retrocaecal position, for instance, rigidity is often absent, because the caecum is distended with gas, preventing the pressure exerted by hand from reaching the inflamed structure.

Appendix in the pelvis: when appendix lies entirely within the pelvis, usually there is complete absence of abdominal rigidity.

In some instances, deep tenderness can be made out just above and to the right of symphysis pubis; there is very rarely diarrhoea due to contact of the inflamed appendix with the rectum.

In post- ileal position, the appendix lies behind the terminal ileum, and diarrhoea is a marked feature. In maldescended (sub hepatitis), tenderness is in the sub hepatic region.

LESSONS LEARNED

- Negative comments by professional staff can be damaging and complicate issues. They serve neither patients nor professionals.
- Acute appendicitis can be difficult to diagnose correctly. It is important to be opened minded.
- Keep good records.
- Signs and symptoms of acute appendicitis depend on anatomical location of the appendix to a great degree.

Went back to my consultation records, wrote back to the patient, explaining all the circumstances in a professional manner. I did not hear back from him, assumed he was satisfied.

Case study 2

INTRODUCTION

This thirty-nine-year-old man was co-owner of a well-known local supermarket with his partner and operated the business seven days a week, working long hours. He was a smoker, consuming ten cigarettes a day, but did not drink alcohol. He was married with three children and enjoyed a happy family life.

PAST MEDICAL HISTORY

The patient had a history of a partial thyroidectomy for a large thyroid enlargement five years previously but was otherwise healthy, took no regular medications, and had no known allergies.

SYMPTOMS

On Boxing Day, at around 6 am, he opened his supermarket as usual. After running the business for about 45 minutes, he had a black coffee and a slice of cake left over from the previous day, which had been stored in the fridge. Shortly afterward, he began to feel unwell and experienced a general sense of malaise. He informed his shop assistant that he was leaving to go home due to feeling poorly, declining both an offer to be taken to the hospital and assistance in driving home. He decided to drive himself in his VW Polo, as his home was only half a mile away.

However, within a minute of leaving, he found himself disoriented, having lost his sense of direction. He became unable to speak, with numbness affecting the right side of his body. His car came to a stop on the wrong side of the road. He tried to use his phone but was unable to communicate. Fortunately, a couple passing by, who were regular customers, recognised him and helped. He handed them his phone, and they promptly called 999, staying with him until the ambulance arrived five minutes later. He was taken to the local hospital.

EXAMINATION

On arrival, his condition was stable, and all examinations were unremarkable. He stayed in the hospital for two days, undergoing MRI and CT scans, as well as blood tests, all of which returned normal results. The consultant discussed the case with him, explaining that no abnormalities were found and that they were unable to provide a clear diagnosis. The patient was discharged with instructions to contact the hospital if any new symptoms arose.

Two days later, the patient visited the practice with his hospital discharge letter, feeling well, but still confused about the incident. During a conversation with his partner about the episode, it emerged that his partner had also felt unwell after eating a slice of the same cake but had gone to bed and recovered. This prompted the patient to contact the customer who had gifted the cake on Christmas Day. Upon inquiry, the customer revealed that the cake was homemade for special occasions and contained cannabis.

DIFFERENTIAL DIAGNOSIS

- Transient ischemic attack (TIA): While the symptoms were consistent with a TIA, the patient had no risk factors such as hypertension, ischemic heart disease, valvular heart disease, congenital heart disease, or carotid bruits. Peripheral pulses were normal, making this diagnosis less likely.

- Viral episode: The sudden onset of symptoms without any fever or other signs of viral infection made this unlikely.
- Drug-induced episode: The patient denied taking any illicit drugs or medications, which initially ruled this out. However, the new information regarding cannabis in the cake raised the possibility of drug-induced symptoms.
- Mental health issues: The patient had no history of psychosis or neurosis, and there were no signs of schizophrenia or depression, making a mental health cause unlikely.
- Exhaustion: Although the patient worked long hours, exhaustion did not explain the slurred speech, numbness, confusion or disorientation.

DIAGNOSIS

The case presents a dilemma, with no clear medical explanation based on conventional investigations. However, the discovery of cannabis in the cake raises the possibility that the symptoms were due to cannabis intoxication, which could account for the neurological and cognitive effects experienced by the patient.

LESSON LEARNED

In some cases, even thorough medical investigations may leave us with unresolved dilemmas. The possibility of drug-induced symptoms from unexpected sources, such as food, should be considered when the clinical picture does not fit conventional diagnoses.

Case study 3

INTRODUCTION

This patient, a twenty-eight-year-old Caucasian female, originally from the Midlands, was a graduate student at a local university. She did not smoke or regularly consume alcohol.

PAST MEDICAL HISTORY

The patient had complained of persistent headaches, but was otherwise healthy, with no history of migraines or significant medical issues. She described her headaches as moderate in intensity, occurring several times a week, and characterised by a throbbing sensation primarily localised to the right side of her head.

SYMPTOMS

On a rainy evening in October, I was working an evening shift at the out-of-hours (OOH) clinic when I received a call to assess this patient. She had reported a sudden worsening of her headache, accompanied by nausea and minimal sensitivity to light, which prompted her to seek medical attention.

Upon her arrival at the clinic, the patient appeared anxious but was otherwise well-nourished and hydrated. She recounted that the headaches had progressively intensified over the past month, often triggered by stress or lack of sleep. This episode, however, had started abruptly that afternoon, disrupting her plans to study for an upcoming exam.

EXAMINATION

During the consultation, I conducted a thorough history and

examination. The patient described her headache as a unilateral, pulsating pain, rated at 8/10 in intensity. She reported associated symptoms of nausea but denied any vomiting, visual disturbances or neurological deficits. Importantly, she had no prior history of similar severe headaches.

Her vital signs were stable: blood pressure was 118/76 mmHg, heart rate was 72 beats per minute (regular), and her temperature was 37.0°C. Neurological examination revealed no focal deficits, and her pupils were equal and reactive to light, no neck stiffness or papilledema.

Palpation of the scalp and neck revealed mild tenderness without any stiffness. There were no signs of systemic illness, such as fever or rash. A focused assessment did not reveal any concerning findings that would necessitate immediate imaging or intervention.

TREATMENT (INITIAL)

Based on the presentation, diagnosed the patient with a probable migraine headache, considering the episodic nature and associated symptoms. provided reassurance, explaining that while her symptoms were distressing, there were no immediate signs of serious underlying pathology, such as a subarachnoid haemorrhage or intracranial mass.

Advised her to manage her pain with over-the-counter analgesics, recommended lifestyle modifications to reduce stress, and encouraged adequate hydration. Additionally, suggested keeping a headache diary to identify potential triggers and noted that she could come back at any time if things get worse.

SUBSEQUENT DEVELOPMENTS

Two weeks later, I received a formal complaint from the patient. After our consultation, her headaches continued unabated, leading her to seek further evaluation at the local emergency department, where she underwent a CT scan. The results indicated the presence of a small intracranial lesion, which required follow-up with a neurologist for further management.

Was taken aback by the complaint, as I believed my assessment and management plan adhered to standard clinical practice. However, two key factors may have contributed to the patient's dissatisfaction:

- Patient misunderstanding: The patient may not have fully understood the nature of her condition or the limitations of my initial diagnosis. Headaches, particularly migraines, can often be subjective and complex, making them challenging to assess and diagnose accurately during a single encounter.
- Delayed diagnosis: The subsequent discovery of the intracranial lesion understandably heightened the patient's concern. She may have perceived my initial assessment as inadequate, feeling that her condition warranted more urgent investigation.

DIAGNOSTIC COMPLEXITY

The evaluation of headaches can be multifaceted, as they can arise from various causes ranging from benign to life-threatening conditions. Key considerations include:

- Migraine vs. secondary headache: It can be challenging to differentiate between primary headaches, such as migraines or tension-type headaches, and secondary headaches due to more serious underlying conditions, like tumours or vascular anomalies.

- Alarm symptoms: Certain red flags, including sudden onset, changes in headache pattern, or neurological symptoms, necessitate further investigation. In this case, the acute change in the patient's headache pattern should have prompted a more cautious approach.
- Diagnostic tools: While physical examination and clinical history are essential, imaging studies like CT or MRI can be critical in ambiguous cases, especially when there are concerning features.

LESSONS LEARNED

- Effective communication: Clear explanations regarding the nature of headache disorders and the rationale behind clinical decisions can help manage patient expectations and reduce misunderstandings.
- Thorough evaluation: It is vital to conduct a comprehensive evaluation and remain vigilant for potential red flags that could indicate secondary causes of headaches.
- Follow-up: Encouraging patients to seek timely follow-up if their symptoms persist or worsen is essential for ensuring ongoing care and proper management.

In light of the complaint, I reviewed my consultation notes and crafted a formal response to the patient, clarifying the circumstances of her initial assessment and expressing empathy for her experience. I have not received further communication from her, leading me to assume that my response addressed her concerns. This case underscores the complexities of headache diagnosis and the necessity of maintaining an open line of communication with patients to facilitate better understanding and satisfaction.

Case study 4

This forty-five-year-old male Caucasian, working as an accountant in Midlands, presented with sudden onset of chest pain. The patient, a non-smoker with a history of occasional social drinking, led a generally active lifestyle, walking regularly and maintaining a healthy diet.

PAST MEDICAL HISTORY

The patient had no significant past medical history apart from mild hypertension, which was well controlled with medication, Amlodipine 5 mg o d

SYMPTOMS

One cold December night, while I was on an out-of-hours (OOH) night shift, I received a call from the central office at 3 am, reporting a patient with sudden chest pain in a city suburb, approximately seven miles from the city centre. The roads were icy, and the weather conditions were treacherous, but I made my way cautiously to the patient's home.

Upon arrival, found the patient sitting on the edge of his bed, appearing anxious and slightly diaphoretic. He described the pain as a tight, squeezing sensation in the centre of his chest, radiating to his left arm, which had started about an hour earlier while he was watching TV. He denied shortness of breath, nausea, or sweating prior to the pain but mentioned a slight feeling of indigestion after eating dinner earlier that evening.

EXAMINATION

The patient appeared well overall but visibly concerned. His vital signs were within normal limits: blood pressure was 130/80 mmHg, pulse was 76 beats per minute (regular), and his temperature was 36.8°C. His respiratory rate was normal, and he was breathing comfortably, without signs of distress.

I conducted a thorough cardiovascular and respiratory examination. There were no abnormal heart sounds, murmurs, or irregular rhythms detected. Lung auscultation revealed clear breath sounds bilaterally. His chest was non-tender on palpation and there were no signs of swelling or redness in his extremities that might suggest deep vein thrombosis.

The patient's pain was atypical for a cardiac origin, as it was not worsened by exertion, and he had no associated symptoms such as sweating, dizziness or nausea that would typically accompany a myocardial infarction. His history of mild indigestion following dinner, combined with the lack of alarming features, led me to suspect that the pain was likely non-cardiac in origin, possibly related to acid reflux or musculoskeletal strain.

TREATMENT (INITIAL)

After the examination, I explained to the patient that while his chest pain was concerning, the absence of typical red flags for a heart attack made a cardiac cause less likely. I suspected his pain could be due to gastroesophageal reflux disease (GERD) or muscle strain, but I recommended keeping a close watch on his symptoms.

I advised him to take an over-the-counter antacid and rest, explaining that if the pain worsened, persisted, or was accompanied by any additional symptoms (such as shortness of breath or sweating), he should immediately seek medical attention. Both the patient and his wife appeared reassured by my explanation, and he agreed to monitor his condition closely.

SUBSEQUENT DEVELOPMENTS

Three days later, I received a formal complaint from the patient's wife. She stated that the following morning, the patient experienced worsening chest pain and decided to visit the emergency department, where he underwent an electrocardiogram (ECG) and blood tests. Normal troponin levels suggest a probable diagnosis of unstable angina. He was admitted to the hospital and underwent angioplasty to clear a partially blocked coronary artery.

I received a formal complaint. I felt I had conducted a thorough assessment and offered reasonable advice based on the patient's presentation at the time.

Two factors may have contributed to the complaint:

- Misjudgement of initial symptoms: Chest pain can be difficult to assess, particularly when it presents atypically. The patient's description of a squeezing sensation, while concerning, lacked many of the classic features of a myocardial infarction (such as radiation to the jaw, profuse sweating or shortness of breath). Despite this, I now realise that even vague or mild chest pain can indicate serious underlying cardiovascular issues and should be investigated more urgently.
- Delayed diagnosis: The patient's symptoms later escalated, resulting in a diagnosis of unstable angina. While my initial evaluation did not reveal any significant abnormalities, the delayed worsening of his condition underscores the challenge of chest pain assessment and the need for a more

cautious approach, particularly in patients with risk factors like hypertension.

DIAGNOSTIC COMPLEXITY

Chest pain is a common but complex symptom with a wide range of potential causes, both cardiac and non-cardiac. The challenge lies in identifying serious conditions early on while avoiding unnecessary alarm for benign causes.

- Cardiac causes: Conditions such as unstable angina, myocardial infarction, and aortic dissection must always be considered in patients presenting with chest pain, especially if they have risk factors such as hypertension, diabetes or a family history of heart disease.
- Non-cardiac causes: Many cases of chest pain are due to non-cardiac issues like gastroesophageal reflux disease (GERD), musculoskeletal strain, or anxiety. These causes often present with similar symptoms but typically lack the severity or systemic signs of cardiac events.
- Alarm symptoms: Sudden, severe pain, pain radiating to the arm, neck, or jaw, and associated symptoms like shortness of breath, sweating, or dizziness should always prompt further investigation, even in the absence of typical risk factors.

LESSONS LEARNED

- Caution in chest pain: Even when chest pain presents without clear cardiac features, it is important to err on the side of caution. In retrospect, recommending an immediate ECG or referral to the emergency department may have provided greater reassurance and allowed for an earlier diagnosis.

- Communication is key: A detailed explanation of the potential risks and the importance of follow-up in cases of chest pain can help ensure patients and their families are vigilant about worsening symptoms.
- Timely investigation: In cases where chest pain persists or seems atypical, early referral for further testing (such as an ECG or blood tests) can prevent delayed diagnoses and ensure prompt treatment.

CONCLUSION

After reviewing the consultation notes, I responded to the patient's complaint with a detailed explanation of the circumstances and an expression of empathy for his experience. In my response, acknowledged the difficulty of diagnosing chest pain accurately and emphasised the importance of early investigation. I have not received further communication from the patient.

Case study 5

INTRODUCTION

The patient was a thirty-six-year-old female who worked as a teacher.

PAST MEDICAL HISTORY

The patient had no known history of TB or recent travel to high-risk areas. She complained of recurrent episodes of abdominal pain and weight loss over the past six months. She had intermittent fever, fatigue and altered bowel habits (diarrhoea alternating with constipation).

SYMPTOMS

The primary complaint was persistent lower abdominal pain, especially in the right iliac fossa, associated with bloating and weight loss. She also had mild fever, general malaise and occasional night sweats. She had no vomiting or significant rectal bleeding.

EXAMINATION

There were no palpable masses, her spleen and liver were not palpable. There was mild tenderness on deep palpation in the ileocaecal region.

I first arranged blood tests; results showed mild anaemia and slightly elevated ESR and CRP, suggestive of an inflammatory process.

Stool tests: Negative for ova, parasites, and bacterial pathogens. Ultrasound of the abdomen: Mild thickening of the terminal ileum and caecum, but inconclusive.

What was the differential diagnosis?

- Malignancy (right sided colon cancer, Appendiceal tumour)
- Crohn's disease, abdominal TB
- Ovarian cancer, abscess, endometriosis
- Diverticular disease
- Renal TB

TREATMENT (INITIAL)

The patient was started on symptomatic treatment, including analgesics and antibiotics for presumed bacterial enterocolitis. No further immediate investigation was pursued.

SUBSEQUENT DEVELOPMENTS

Over the next few weeks, the patient's symptoms persisted. She developed more severe weight loss and occasional blood-streaked stool. The abdominal pain became more localised to the right iliac fossa.

A repeat ultrasound and CT scan of the abdomen suggested ileocecal thickening, but still no specific diagnosis.

SUBSEQUENT TREATMENT

A colonoscopy was eventually performed which revealed ulceration and nodularity at the ileocaecal junction; a biopsy was taken.

What do think the most likely diagnosis was?

The initial non-specific findings led to a delay in diagnosing ileocaecal TB. The biopsy results from colonoscopy eventually confirmed granulomatous inflammation consistent with tuberculosis. PCR testing confirmed the presence of Mycobacterium tuberculosis.

A Mantoux test was also positive, and a chest X-ray showed old, healed TB lesions, further supporting the diagnosis.

TREATMENT

- Antitubercular therapy (ATT): The patient was started on a four-drug ATT regimen (Isoniazid, Rifampicin, Pyrazinamide, and Ethambutol) for six to nine months.
- Nutritional support: To address malnutrition from weight loss.
- Follow-up: Regular monitoring of liver function due to the hepatotoxicity risk of TB medications.

LESSONS LEARNED

- Ileocaecal TB, though rare in non-endemic regions, should be considered in the differential diagnosis of chronic abdominal pain, especially in patients with systemic symptoms like weight loss and fever.
- Early endoscopic evaluation and biopsy can significantly reduce delays in diagnosis.
- Misdiagnosis or delayed diagnosis can lead to complications, including intestinal obstruction, perforation, or fistula formation.

This case highlights the importance of considering TB in gastrointestinal cases with chronic abdominal symptoms, even in non-endemic areas, to avoid diagnostic delays and ensure timely management.

This structure emphasises the diagnostic process, the initial misinterpretation and the eventual confirmation of TB, showcasing the critical need for a thorough differential diagnosis in cases of chronic abdominal symptoms.

Case study 6

INTRODUCTION

The patient, who had immigrated from the Middle East thirty years previously, was a seventy-eight-year-old retired factory worker (he had retired at sixty-five). He lived with his wife and daughter in a private terrace house. He smoked one pack of cigarettes per day until the age of sixty-five and consumed around ten pints of alcohol per week.

SYMPTOMS

Five weeks post-retirement, the patient developed an upper respiratory tract infection.

He attended the practice with symptoms of wheezing, minimal shortness of breath, a runny nose, and excessive coughing. No haemoptysis noted.

PAST MEDICAL HISTORY

Overall, the patient had been in relatively good health. He had well-controlled hypertension (on amlodipine). He had a urethral stricture (previously treated with urethral dilatation), scheduled for another dilatation in three weeks; allergy to penicillin; use of a salbutamol inhaler as needed.

EXAMINATION

The patient appeared well and was accompanied by his concerned wife.

He had no evident shortness of breath or wheezing. Oxygen saturation was 98%, temperature was 37.5°C, pulse 90 bpm, and BP 140/73 mmHg.

Mild expiratory wheeze noted bilaterally, with no signs of central cyanosis or heart failure. A soft systolic murmur was detected in the left lateral chest area. JVP was normal, and the remainder of the examination was unremarkable.

DIAGNOSIS AND INITIAL TREATMENT

Treated as viral upper respiratory tract infection. Advice was given to take paracetamol, maintain hydration, and monitor symptoms. The patient went home satisfied, but went to A&E a few days later, as his condition did not improve. He was prescribed clarithromycin 500 mg twice daily for one week. He subsequently improved and underwent urethral dilatation without complications.

SUBSEQUENT DEVELOPMENT

Three weeks later, the patient reported feeling fatigued and easily exhausted with minimal effort, but without any other specific symptoms.
Pulse: 100 bpm, regular.
Temperature: 37.5°C.
Chest and throat clear.
Urine analysis: No abnormalities.
The diagnosis was likely to be viral infection. He was reassured, advised to take pain relief, and instructed to return if needed.

Subsequent discharge letters from A&E indicated the patient had attended three times, each time being sent home with painkillers. Basic blood tests conducted during those visits were normal.

FURTHER SYMPTOMS AND SUBSEQUENT TREATMENT

Two weeks later, the patient returned with persistent fatigue and new onset of night sweats.
Temperature: 38°C.
Pulse: 106 bpm, regular.
Urine analysis: blood and protein detected.

Given the persistence of symptoms, including night sweats and abnormal urine findings, there was concern that something more serious was underlying the patient's condition.

Blood tests and chest X-ray were requested, with the following results
ESR: 70 mm/hr.
CRP: 55 mg/L.
Haemoglobin: 10 g/dL (normochromic, normocytic anaemia).
Renal and liver function: normal.

The patient was contacted and asked to return to the practice. After reviewing the blood results, the patient was referred to the on-call medical team and admitted to the medical ward for further evaluation.

WHAT DO THINK THE DIFFERENTIAL DIAGNOSIS AT THAT TIME?

Renal TB
Renal malignancy (Hypernephroma)
Bacterial endocarditis

THE PATIENT'S PRESENTATION INCLUDED:

- Persistent fatigue and night sweats.
- Microscopic haematuria and proteinuria.
- Elevated inflammatory markers (ESR and CRP).
- Normochromic, normocytic anaemia.
- Previous heart murmur.
- Recent minor urological procedure (urethral dilatation), a possible source of bacterial entry.

DIAGNOSIS

While symptoms were non-specific, the combination of these factors pointed towards a diagnosis of infective endocarditis.

Infective endocarditis typically has an insidious onset and can take months to diagnose. It primarily affects damaged valves (e.g. mitral and aortic valves) or prosthetic valves. In drug users, it may affect the tricuspid valve. Post-mortem findings often reveal infarctions of the spleen or kidneys. Late-stage signs include petechial haemorrhages on the skin and mucous membranes, nail splinter haemorrhages, and Osler's nodes (tender nodules on the fingertips). Emboli may lead to strokes or myocardial infarctions.

LESSONS LEARNED

- Persistent unexplained fever, especially with non-specific symptoms, should prompt reassessment of heart valves.
- Delayed diagnosis can significantly affect patient outcomes.
- Early signs of endocarditis are subtle; later signs can be life-threatening.
- Prophylactic antibiotics are critical for patients undergoing minor surgical procedures if they have known heart valve disease.

- Patients with heart valve conditions should carry identification cards to inform medical personnel of their condition.

Endocarditis remains a serious condition, often fatal if untreated.

Case study 7

Though I wasn't directly involved in this case, I found it particularly interesting, offering valuable lessons for clinical practice.

INTRODUCTION

A thirty-two-year-old Egyptian man, employed as a teacher in Libya for the past three years, presented with a complex medical history. Married with two children, he had never smoked nor consumed alcohol.

I first met the patient in London during a busy summer, when the city was bustling with tourists, making it rare to encounter locals. Many individuals from the Middle East seek medical treatment in the UK, and this gentleman was no exception. He had travelled to London to consult a physician recommended by his contacts in Libya. Lacking proficiency in English, we assisted him in locating the doctor's office and accompanied him to the consultation, acting as an interpreter.

SYMPTOMS

The patient had been treated previously in Tripoli by a cardiologist for recurrent palpitations and dizziness, symptoms he had experienced intermittently over several years. He was on propranolol (a beta-blocker) but reported no other medical conditions or allergies.

EXAMINATION

While the examination details are limited, I can note that he appeared generally well, with no signs of shortness of breath. His approximate weight was 75 kg, and his height was 175 cm.

There was clearly some crucial information missing that would be helpful in making a diagnosis. This related to family history. The patient disclosed that his mother had died suddenly at the age of forty, and his brother had also died suddenly at the age of five. Both deaths were unexplained, pointing towards a potential genetic or familial condition.

What was the diagnosis with positive family history of premature death?

HYPERTROPHIC OBSTRUCTIVE CARDIOMYOPATHY (HOCM)

In many cases, myocardial disease may be part of a broader systemic disorder, with varying degrees of cardiac involvement. Conditions such as haemochromatosis, sarcoidosis, amyloidosis, uraemia, muscular dystrophies, and connective tissue disorders can all affect the heart. Cardiomyopathy is also associated with alcoholism and, in rare cases, late-stage pregnancy.

In cases where no systemic disorder is identified, and no specific causative agent is found, a family history often provides critical clues. This was the case here, where the family history of sudden death raised concerns about an underlying inherited condition.

- Congestive cardiomyopathy: this is the most common form, characterised by cardiomegaly, valvular regurgitation and progressive left-sided heart failure, eventually involving the right side.
- Hypertrophic cardiomyopathy (HOCM): this form is marked

by significant thickening of the interventricular septum, which can obstruct the outflow from the left ventricle, creating a clinical picture like aortic stenosis. Although the exact cause is often unclear, a family history is frequently observed.

OTHER RARE FORMS OF CARDIOMYOPATHY INCLUDE:

- Restrictive cardiomyopathy, which mimics constrictive pericarditis.
- Obliterative cardiomyopathy commonly seen in tropical regions, such as endomyocardial fibrosis.
- Arrhythmias are a common feature in all types of cardiomyopathies and are a leading cause of sudden death, particularly in cases of HOCM.
- The diagnosis of cardiomyopathy should be considered when there is unexplained cardiomegaly or unresponsive heart failure. Major causes of heart disease, such as rheumatic, hypertensive, ischaemic, thyrotoxic, or congenital conditions, should be excluded first. An echocardiogram is the primary diagnostic tool for confirming HOCM.

LESSONS LEARNED

- The critical importance of family history in diagnosing certain diseases.
- Arrhythmia is a common cause of sudden death in HOCM.
- Cardiomyopathy should be suspected in any case of unexplained cardiomegaly or refractory congestive heart failure.
- Echocardiography is the investigation of choice for diagnosing HOCM.

Case study 8

INTRODUCTION

The patient was a thirty-five-year-old Caucasian female, married, mother of two children (aged seven and four). She was a non-smoker, consumed alcohol socially and worked as a graphic designer. She had a history of heavy and painful periods but has never had any significant medical issues otherwise.

SYMPTOMS

I saw the patient at an out-of-hours (OOH) clinic on a rainy Saturday evening in March. The waiting room was moderately busy, filled with patients dealing with a variety of complaints. When I called her in, she walked in slowly, wincing with each step. Her face was pale, and she seemed fatigued, as though she had been coping with severe pain for some time.

She explained that she had been experiencing worsening lower abdominal pain for the past six months, but over the last two weeks, it had become unbearable. The pain was cyclical, typically worse during her periods, but now it persisted throughout her cycle. She described the pain as a deep, stabbing sensation, radiating to her lower back and thighs. She had been taking ibuprofen and paracetamol to manage the discomfort, but these were no longer effective.

Her periods had always been heavy and painful, but recently, they had become even more debilitating, accompanied by severe bloating, nausea, and occasional constipation. She had also noticed pain during intercourse, something she had never experienced before. She felt exhausted, emotionally drained, and was finding it increasingly difficult to manage her daily responsibilities, both at work and at home.

INITIAL TREATMENT

Her GP had prescribed stronger painkillers and advised her to try hormonal contraceptives to regulate her periods. However, the pain persisted, and the contraceptives made her feel nauseous and bloated, leading her to discontinue them after just two months. Despite several visits to the GP and the use of pain relief, she felt like she was being dismissed, with her symptoms attributed to "stress" or "just part of being a woman".

EXAMINATION

She appeared visibly distressed and fatigued. On palpation, her lower abdomen was tender, especially in the pelvic region, but there were no signs of acute peritonitis. Her vital signs were stable, with a temperature of 37°C, pulse 90 bpm (sinus rhythm), blood pressure 110/70, and oxygen saturation of 98%. A pelvic examination revealed significant tenderness along the pelvic floor and adnexa, but there was no obvious mass.

I recommended an urgent referral to a gynaecologist for further investigation, including a pelvic ultrasound and possible laparoscopy, also advised her to maintain a pain diary, tracking the timing and severity of her symptoms in relation to her menstrual cycle, to provide more detailed information to the specialist. I contact her GP, who responded positively.

What was most likely diagnosis?

A month later, the patient underwent a diagnostic laparoscopy, which confirmed the presence of endometriosis, with lesions found on her ovaries, pelvic ligaments and along the bowel. The gynaecologist explained that endometriosis occurs when tissue like the lining of the uterus grows outside the uterine cavity, causing inflammation, scarring and chronic pain. Her condition had likely been developing for years but had not been recognised.

Endometriosis is a chronic condition where tissue like the endometrium (the lining of the uterus) grows in areas outside the uterus, such as the ovaries, fallopian tubes, and the pelvic lining. This ectopic tissue responds to the hormonal changes of the menstrual cycle, leading to inflammation, pain, and the formation of scar tissue. The condition can cause a range of symptoms, from mild discomfort to debilitating pain, and is one of the leading causes of infertility.

Patients often experience chronic pelvic pain, heavy menstrual bleeding, painful intercourse, and bowel or urinary symptoms, though the severity of symptoms does not always correlate with the extent of the disease. Unfortunately, endometriosis is frequently underdiagnosed or misdiagnosed, as it can present with symptoms like other gynaecological or gastrointestinal disorders. Delayed diagnosis is common, with an average of 7-10 years from the onset of symptoms to a confirmed diagnosis.

LESSONS LEARNED

- Chronic pelvic pain, particularly in young women, should prompt consideration of endometriosis, especially if symptoms worsen during the menstrual cycle.
- Patients with recurring symptoms should be taken seriously, and early referral to a specialist is key to diagnosing

conditions like endometriosis.

- Hormonal therapies and pain management strategies may not be effective for all patients.
- Emphasising the need for individualised treatment plans
- Laparoscopy remains the gold standard for diagnosing endometriosis and assessing the extent of the disease.
- Endometriosis can significantly impact a patient's quality of life, making timely diagnosis and appropriate treatment critical.

Case study 9

INTRODUCTION

This was a forty-two-year-old Caucasian female, married, mother of a five-year-old boy. She had never smoked, drank alcohol occasionally, and had worked as a receptionist at a solicitor's firm for the past decade.

I saw her at an out-of-hours (OOH) clinic one weekend in July. The waiting room was packed with patients of varying ages. As I followed the OOH protocol of prioritising children, I first called in a young child with a suspected insect bite. It was a hot day, and many people had been enjoying the parks, resulting in a surge of insect bite cases.

However, one patient caught my attention—a woman sitting quietly, looking down, supporting her head with her right fist under her chin. After quickly treating the child, I called this woman, who was accompanied by her energetic and cheerful little boy and her husband. Her son, blissfully unaware of the seriousness of his mother's condition, played happily in the consulting room.

SYMPTOMS

She explained that she had been feeling unwell for seventeen days, initially experiencing two episodes of watery diarrhoea and abdominal pain across her entire abdomen. There was no blood in her stools, and she vomited only once. No one else in her family was affected. After two days without improvement, the diarrhoea stopped, but her symptoms worsened, prompting her to visit her GP, who assured her it was likely a self-limiting bug that would resolve on its own.

However, over the next few days, her condition deteriorated. She returned to her GP twice more and visited the OOH service twice as well. She reported losing her appetite and shedding weight at a rate of one pound per day. Frustrated, she added, "Now I am feeling very ill, and nobody is taking me seriously."

PAST MEDICAL HISTORY

Her medical history was unremarkable - no known allergies, no regular medication and no prior health issues other than taking paracetamol and a short course of painkillers for mild back pain.

EXAMINATION

On examination, she appeared pale and mildly dehydrated, with a temperature of 38°C, a pulse of 115 (sinus rhythm), blood pressure of 90/60, and oxygen saturation of 96%. There were no signs of a rash, her abdomen was tender but not rigid, and the rest of the physical exam was unremarkable.

DIAGNOSIS

I suspected she was in a septic state. I kept her in a separate room for observation and immediately called 999. I also informed the emergency department at the local hospital about her condition. The ambulance arrived within five minutes and transported her to the hospital. The underlying cause of the sepsis was unclear at the time.

I called the hospital the next day, but no diagnosis had been made yet. I contacted them again two days later, and still, there was no definitive answer. On the sixth day, I reached out to her partner, who informed me she was undergoing CT and MRI scans. Finally, on the seventh day, a diagnosis was confirmed.

What was the possible diagnosis?

During another out-of-hours session, the receptionist called to inform me that a lady wished to see me, although she was not a patient. I requested a staff member to accompany her, as I wanted to be cautious. The woman entered and asked, "Do you remember me?" I initially did not, but after she reminded me of the events, I recalled her case. She handed me a card and said, "Thank you, plus one."

Ulcerative colitis is an inflammatory bowel disease affecting the colon and the distal foot of the ileum. Its cause is unknown. Early symptoms include watery diarrhoea, occurring day and night, followed by bloody and mucus-filled stools. In 90 per cent of cases, the rectum is affected. The condition can present as acute and fulminant or develop into a chronic form.

Unfortunately, in this case, diagnosis was delayed due to her atypical presentation and repeated visits to the GP and out-of-hours services without recognition of the seriousness of her condition. This case highlights how diseases can present in unexpected ways and the importance of keeping an open mind during diagnosis. Fortunately, the patient did not suffer a perforation.

LESSONS LEARNED

- It is vital to be vigilant for unusual presentations of illnesses. Take multiple patient visits seriously.
- Follow-up cases provide valuable learning opportunities.

- Act swiftly and responsibly when necessary.
- Suspected sepsis requires immediate attention and action.

Case study 10

It was a sunny Sunday afternoon in the summer of 2005 and was working an out-of-hours (OOH) shift. The OOH controller passed on a routine call—a seven-month-old child with a rash, classified as non-urgent and to be seen within six hours. However, as I was nearby, arrived at the home just 30 minutes after receiving the call.

Upon arrival, a young child opened the door, and was greeted by the grandmother, who was sitting beside her daughter. The infant was resting in the grandmother's lap.

SYMPTOMS

Almost immediately, felt something was amiss. The child was blinking rapidly and seemed unable to keep his eyes open in the light. Inquired about the rash, and the grandmother, downplaying the situation, mentioned it was "not very much," just faint red patches on the abdomen, with cold hands and feet.

EXAMINATION

I quickly examined the rash, faint, red, and non-blanching, and could not elicit neck stiffness. The child's temperature was 37.4°C. At this moment, I recognised the gravity of the situation. Suspecting meningococcal meningitis, knew I had to act swiftly.

INITIAL TREATMENT

Asked the mother to immediately call 999. Simultaneously, I retrieved Benzylpenicillin (Penicillin G) from my medical bag, mixed the vial with distilled water, and administered it via injection into the child's right anterolateral thigh. Just four minutes later, the ambulance arrived. I briefed the paramedics on the suspected case of meningococcal meningitis and urged them to take the child to the nearest hospital, which was only a mile away, with minimal traffic due to the Sunday afternoon.

SUBSEQUENT TREATMENT

Later that evening, about six hours after the initial incident, I contacted the hospital for an update. The paediatric consultant informed me that while the child was being transferred from A&E to the paediatric ward, he deteriorated. Unfortunately, there was no ventilator available, and the decision was made to airlift the child by helicopter to a hospital 40 miles away for further treatment.

A week later, followed up with the family. They were relieved to report that the child was doing well, breathing without mechanical support, and expected to be discharged soon. The diagnosis of meningococcal meningitis was confirmed.

LESSONS LEARNED

- Always be cautious, especially when information is limited or incomplete.
- Carrying emergency medication, like Benzylpenicillin, in your medical bag is crucial—it can save lives.
- When faced with a suspected serious illness, avoid unnecessary and time-consuming examinations. Focus only on what is clinically relevant.
- Don't hesitate to involve family members for help, such as calling emergency services, while you focus on critical interventions.

- Always contact the hospital ahead of time so they can prepare to handle emergencies appropriately.

Case study 11

INTRODUCTION

A fifty-eight-year-old man, registered with the practice for the past ten years, presented with a significant smoking history, twenty cigarettes a day since the age of twenty. He worked for the city council, was married with two grown children, and lived in a council house with his wife.

SYMPTOMS

The patient rarely attended the surgery, but he came in to see me complaining of pain in his right lower limb. He reported the pain had been ongoing for several months, worsening during walking, and subsiding with rest. Recently, the pain had intensified, reducing his walking ability to just a few yards. He had been unable to work for the past week due to the severity of the symptoms.

PAST MEDICAL HISTORY

The patient had no significant previous medical history, was not on any regular medications, and had no known allergies.

EXAMINATION

On examination, the patient appeared stressed, but was not short of breath at rest, cyanotic or clinically anaemic. His vital signs were stable:
Weight: 71 kg
Height: 177 cm
Temperature: 37°C
Blood pressure: 138/78 mmHg
Pulse: 100 bpm, regular

Cardiovascular examination revealed no cardiomegaly. Heart sounds were normal, with no added sounds detected. Right-sided carotid bruit, loud; left carotid, normal.

Respiratory examination showed an occasional wheeze, which cleared after coughing. No other abnormalities were detected.

The patient appeared anxious, likely due to the unfamiliarity of being ill, but no neurological abnormalities were noted in terms of his central nervous system.

Upper limbs were symmetrical and had no abnormalities. The right hand showed tobacco staining.

On examining the right leg, the foot appeared cyanotic and cold below the knee. Popliteal pulse was absent, and neither the dorsalis pedis nor the posterior tibial pulses were palpable. The femoral pulse was difficult to feel. No ulceration or signs of infection were present.

The left leg was normal in appearance, with all pulses palpable.

The abdomen was soft, with no bruit detected.

DIAGNOSIS AND TREATMENT

Recognised the urgency of the situation, suspecting imminent gangrene in the right lower limb, immediately dictated a referral letter to the hospital and contacted the local emergency department to emphasise the critical nature of the case. The letter was quickly typed, signed and handed to the patient, who was then sent to the hospital.

However, the following morning, the patient returned to the practice. Despite the clear urgency, the hospital had discharged him back to his GP. Concerned, I contacted another hospital, sending the same referral letter. Once again, the patient was discharged, leaving him increasingly stressed and frustrated.

WHAT WOULD BE YOUR ACTION PLAN CURRENTLY?

I could not allow this patient to risk losing his leg. Determined, I contacted yet another hospital, requesting to speak directly to the on-call vascular surgeon. Fortunately, I managed to get two minutes of his time and stressed the severity of the situation. The surgeon agreed to see the patient immediately. I wrote a covering letter with the surgeon's name on the envelope and sent the patient to the hospital.

The following day, I followed up with the same surgeon. He confirmed that I had referred the patient just in time. Had there been further delays, the patient's leg might have been lost. He expressed relief at intervening at the right moment, acknowledging that the leg was saved in the nick of time.

A few days later, the patient returned to the practice to express his gratitude, bringing a box of chocolates for the staff.

This case highlights a common and unfortunate situation in general practice. Hospitals, under significant pressure and often understaffed, may discharge patients inappropriately, leading to potentially severe consequences. In this case, the delays could have resulted in the loss of a limb, which would have been a devastating outcome for both the patient and the healthcare system.

GPs are often caught in a dilemma when faced with clear life-threatening situations. It is our responsibility as primary care providers to ensure our patients receive the best care possible. We cannot simply step back and allow preventable harm to occur.

LESSONS LEARNED

- GPs remain responsible for their patients' care.
- Hospitals may discharge patients inappropriately, even in critical cases. GPs must reassess their patients' needs and

escalate care if necessary.

- In urgent cases, immediate patient care should be the top priority. Once stabilised, any failures in care should be addressed.
- Potentially pursuing formal complaints or further actions against the hospitals involved.

Case study 12

INTRODUCTION

This case occurred at an out-of-hours (OOH) centre, where my involvement was minimal, but I found it particularly interesting due to the serious implications. A few years ago, was working a night shift at the OOH centre, and a twenty-two-year-old woman attended a booked appointment, accompanied by her older sister.

SYMPTOMS

The patient complained of a sore throat that had persisted for a couple of days. As I questioned her, she shared a longer, troubling history regarding her sore throat.

About two weeks prior, she had visited the same OOH centre for a sore throat. After a full assessment, the attending doctor prescribed Penicillin-V tablets, 500mg, to be taken four times daily. She filled the prescription at a local pharmacy and began taking the medication. However, after two days, she began feeling increasingly unwell. Her sister took her back to the OOH, where she was examined by another doctor. He assured her that the medication was appropriate and advised her to continue the treatment.

The following day, her condition worsened, with the development of mouth ulcers and a fever. She returned to the OOH centre, but once again, the doctor advised her to continue taking the same medication. Feeling even worse the next day, she decided to visit the Accident and Emergency (A&E) department at the local hospital. There, she was told it was likely a viral infection, which would improve with time. Frustrated and feeling like she was "fighting against a wall", she demanded a blood test before leaving the hospital. Reluctantly, the hospital ordered a full blood count (FBC).

Shortly thereafter, a consultant haematologist contacted the emergency department, expressing concern about her blood test results. He requested to see the patient immediately, leading to a definitive diagnosis.

What do you think went wrong?

EXAMINATION

I saw the patient a few days later when she came to the OOH centre again, still feeling unwell and with a sore throat. Her past medical history was unremarkable, with no known allergies and no regular medications. On examination, she appeared well. Her vitals were as follows: temperature 37.2°C, pulse 88 bpm, oxygen saturation 98%, and blood pressure 124/78 mmHg. Examination of her throat revealed redness but no pus, and her tonsils appeared normal. Cardiovascular and respiratory examinations were unremarkable. There was no jaundice or lymphadenopathy, but her urine showed protein ++.

TREATMENT

At this point, was unsure how to proceed given the complexity of her situation. I contacted the haematology department and discussed the case with the haematologist on call. Based on their advice, provided the patient with a delayed prescription for amoxicillin, advising her to take it if her symptoms worsened, while keeping her haematology appointment. The patient was satisfied with this plan and left with the prescription.

THE ANSWER:

The patient had been given a prescription for Penicillamine instead of Penicillin. This error occurred due to a computer-generated prescription, where the first doctor mistakenly ticked Penicillamine instead of Penicillin. The prescription was signed without verifying the medication. The pharmacist, who dispensed a very high dose of Penicillamine, should have questioned the prescription, but unfortunately, this did not happen. Over the course of several visits to the OOH centre and the A&E department, the error was repeatedly overlooked, despite the patient's worsening condition.

It was only when the abnormal blood test results prompted the involvement of a haematologist that the error was uncovered. By this point, the patient had experienced significant discomfort and distress, a clear case of clinical neglect across both primary and secondary care.

LESSONS LEARNED

- Always verify prescriptions. Clinicians must carefully
- Review prescriptions after printing and before signing them, especially when generated by computer systems.
- It is essential for clinicians to verify patient medications thoroughly, particularly when there are concerns about treatment efficacy.
- Clinicians should re-evaluate the case if the patient does not improve as expected.
- Multiple visits within a short timeframe should raise red flags, prompting a more detailed investigation of the underlying issue.

Case study 13

INTRODUCTION

While working an overnight shift during a freezing winter in 1990, received a call at 6.15 am Fortunately, the driver was stationed nearby, as we were nearing the end of our shift at 7 am. After quickly locating the address using an A-Z map (in the days before Google maps or mobile phones), we arrived at the patient's home within seven minutes.

The patient's husband greeted us at the door, relieved by our prompt arrival. I introduced myself and obtained additional details about the patient, a forty-seven-year-old woman working as a secretary at a solicitor's firm. She was a non-smoker and a social drinker.

SYMPTOMS

The patient had contacted us due to severe central abdominal pain that had persisted for approximately six hours, along with a single episode of non-bloody vomiting. She had not opened her bowels for twelve hours, could not pass gas and had not eaten outside the home. Her husband and teenage children were unaffected.

The pain had begun suddenly, coming in waves, but did not radiate to her back, nor was it associated with urination. Her last menstrual period had ended a week earlier.

INITIAL TREATMENT

She mentioned that she had experienced similar abdominal pain a few months prior, and her GP had referred her for a barium enema. The radiology report had raised the possibility of a small lesion in the right colon, but no definitive conclusions were drawn. At the time, her symptoms had resolved completely, and after a discussion with her GP, she decided to wait and monitor the situation, reassured by her GP's confidence that nothing serious was likely.

EXAMINATION

Upon examination, the patient appeared comfortable, as her pain was intermittent. There were no signs of anaemia or jaundice. She was approximately 169 cm tall and weighed 65 kg. Her vital signs were as follows: temperature 36.9°C, pulse 100 bpm (sinus rhythm), and blood pressure 135/84 mmHg.

Abdominal examination revealed no distension, masses, or hepatomegaly. There was some discomfort in the right and mid-abdomen, but no tenderness or rebound tenderness. Cardiovascular and respiratory examinations were unremarkable. Bowel sounds were loud, suggesting increased peristaltic activity.

A) What do you think the diagnosis was?
B) What would be your action plan at that time?

Given the patient's inability to pass gas, the loud bowel sounds, and her history of a prior inconclusive barium enema suggesting a possible lesion, I was concerned about the likelihood of bowel obstruction. Immediately contacted the nearest hospital and emphasised the urgency of the case. I provided a detailed letter for the surgical team and arranged for an ambulance to transport the patient to the hospital without delay.

Within minutes, the ambulance arrived. The crew efficiently loaded the patient, and she was on her way to the hospital, leaving behind her anxious children who still had to prepare for school.

DIFFERENTIAL DIAGNOSIS

This case presented as an acute abdomen with a broad differential diagnosis, including pancreatitis, appendicitis, gallbladder stones, Crohn's disease, ulcerative colitis, mesenteric ischaemia, volvulus, and intussusception. However, several key factors pointed towards bowel obstruction. The patient's inability to pass gas was a significant indicator, supported by the presence of loud bowel sounds. Additionally, her prior barium study raised suspicion of a lesion, which played a critical role in interpreting the current findings.

Conditions like pancreatitis were less likely due to the lack of generalised abdominal tenderness and systemic symptoms. Appendicitis and gallbladder disease were also considered but deemed unlikely based on the pain's location and the absence of jaundice or tenderness in specific areas.

The final diagnosis was right-sided colon cancer with bowel obstruction.

TREATMENT

Two days later, I contacted the on-call surgeon from that night. He confirmed that the patient had been taken directly to the operating theatre, where a tumour was discovered in the right colon. The growth was successfully removed, and the patient was stabilised in the surgical ward.

LESSONS LEARNED

- Inability to pass gas in the context of acute abdominal pain may be a critical sign of bowel obstruction.
- Swift and responsible action, including arranging for immediate transport, can prevent severe complications and improve outcomes.
- Suspicious findings in radiology reports should never be ignored, as they can provide early clues to life-threatening conditions.

Case study 14

INTRODUCTION

A forty-four-year-old married male, a non-smoker, who consumed approximately fourteen pints of alcohol per week, presented to the clinic with concerns after a conversation with a friend at the pub. The patient, who had worked for British Gas for the previous twenty years, lived with his wife and twelve-year-old child in a private residence.

SYMPTOMS

The patient had noticed muscle wasting in both hands, specifically over the last three weeks, without any associated pain. His friend suggested he see a GP after mentioning that a relative had a similar issue and was referred to the hospital.

The patient returned from a one-month holiday in Spain three weeks prior, where he enjoyed the warm weather with his family. He reported no numbness, loss of sensation, weight loss, cough, haemoptysis, or urinary issues. His appetite remained good. The patient's past medical history included two episodes of back pain, successfully managed with simple analgesia, and seasonal hay fever, for which he took cetirizine as needed. He had no known allergies, though he suspected a possible pollen allergy.

EXAMINATION

The patient looked well, non-anaemic, no shortness of breath.
Weight 72 kg, height 179 cm, BP 130/74.

Cardiovascular system: No cardiomegaly, normal heart sounds.

Respiratory system: No clubbing, normal chest shape, normal breath sounds.

On examining the patient's upper limbs, I found bilateral muscle wasting in the hands, most prominently in the thenar and hypothenar eminences, including the dorsum of the hands. Grip strength was good, with no joint swelling, full range of motion and no pain. Sensation was slightly reduced in all modalities in both hands. Coordination and reflexes were normal. Elbow and shoulder power were preserved.

Lower limbs were symmetrical in shape and length, with no muscle wasting or fasciculations, normal reflexes and power. Plantar reflexes were normal.

Neurological: Romberg's sign was negative and cranial nerve examination was unremarkable.

After discussion with the patient, I arranged for the following investigations:

Full blood count (FBC)
Erythrocyte sedimentation rate (ESR)
Liver function tests (LFTs)
Renal function tests
Vitamin B12 and folate levels
Chest X-ray

The patient attended a follow-up appointment 10 days later, at which point all tests, including radiological imaging, were normal. The patient reported no improvement in his symptoms.

Given the normal test results and the lack of a clear diagnosis, I felt it necessary to seek specialist input. I dictated a referral letter to a local neurologist, asking for a consultation at the earliest opportunity.

What do you think the likely diagnosis was?

DIFFERENTIAL DIAGNOSIS

Different diagnoses were feasible: peripheral neuropathy; trauma; age-related atrophy; malnutrition;
osteoarthritis of the hands; motor neurone disease; rheumatoid arthritis;
ulnar and median nerve compression;
other potential causes.

Despite this differential list, none of the conditions satisfactorily explained the patient's presentation.

SUBSEQUENT DEVELOPMENTS

A month later, the patient returned to the clinic with correspondence from the hospital. The neurologist initially struggled to pinpoint the diagnosis but delved deeper into the patient's history, particularly his recent holiday in Spain. Upon further discussion, it emerged that the patient had hired a motorbike during his vacation and spent considerable time using it daily.

The neurologist concluded that excessive use of the motorbike, with jerky movements, likely led to ulnar and median nerve compression, explaining the muscle wasting in both hands. This condition is expected to improve, though nerve recovery can be slow.

The patient was reassured, and no further investigations were deemed necessary. A follow-up appointment was scheduled for six months.

LESSONS LEARNED

- It is important to seek specialist help when uncertain about a diagnosis.
- A detailed history is critical for identifying the underlying cause of symptoms.

Case study 15

INTRODUCTION

The patient was a healthy two-year-old girl The child was full-term, born via vaginal delivery to non-smoking professional parents. Both parents consumed alcohol socially. Her immunisations were up-to-date, and she had no significant past medical history.

SYMPTOMS

On a Sunday morning, the child developed a fever without any noticeable respiratory or gastrointestinal symptoms. The parents administered paracetamol, which temporarily improved her condition, but the fever recurred. The temperature reached 39°C, prompting the parents to call the emergency services for a home visit.

EXAMINATION AND INITIAL TREATMENT

The attending doctor, after examination, diagnosed a viral upper respiratory tract infection and advised continued paracetamol every six hours.

However, the child's fever persisted, accompanied by rapid breathing and poor oral intake, though there was no cough, runny nose or diarrhoea. On Monday morning, the concerned parents sought an urgent appointment.

FURTHER EXAMINATION

On examination, the child was tachypnoeic, with a respiratory rate of 30 breaths per minute, a pulse of 144 bpm, and a temperature of 39°C. There were no signs of cyanosis or neck stiffness. Chest auscultation revealed right-sided posterior crepitations without wheezing. The remainder of the examination was unremarkable. The working diagnosis was pneumonia, and a referral was made to the local paediatric unit. The child was taken to the hospital by the parents, where the diagnosis of lobar pneumonia was confirmed.

Three weeks later, the child presented again with similar symptoms, including high fever and shortness of breath. She was promptly referred to the hospital, where she was again diagnosed with right-sided lobar pneumonia and admitted for one week. A third episode occurred a few weeks later, also diagnosed as right-sided lobar pneumonia.

Following the third recurrence, the parents sought a second opinion due to their concerns about the repeated episodes. A referral was made to the respiratory team at a children's hospital in Birmingham. The respiratory registrar provided insight into the possible underlying cause, and the child was seen in the clinic the next day. Following the hospital's further evaluation, was treated and sent home, the child did not experience any further episodes of pneumonia.

What was the diagnosis?

DIFFERENTIAL DIAGNOSIS:

There are number of different causes of recurrent lobar pneumonia.

- Aspiration syndrome. Recurrent aspiration, possibly due to swallowing difficulties or gastroesophageal reflux, may cause repeated lung infections, particularly in the right lower lobe due to its anatomical structure.
- Pulmonary anomalies or structural abnormalities. Congenital malformations, such as bronchial atresia, sequestration, or

cystic adenomatoid malformation, could predispose the child to recurrent infections localised to a specific lobe.

- congenital heart disease. Conditions like a left-to-right shunt may lead to pulmonary over circulation and predispose the child to recurrent pneumonia.
- Sickle cell disease. Although less common in certain populations, sickle cell disease can lead to acute chest syndrome or recurrent lung infections.
- Cystic fibrosis though unlikely, given the lack of significant cough or gastrointestinal symptoms, should be considered in any child with recurrent pneumonia due to thick mucus plugging and infections.
- Primary ciliary dyskinesia. This condition impairs mucociliary clearance, leading to recurrent respiratory infections, often involving the same region of the lungs.
- A retained foreign body in the right bronchus could cause localized infection and inflammation, leading to recurrent pneumonia in the same lobe.
- An underlying immune system disorder, such as primary immunodeficiency, could lead to recurrent bacterial infections, including pneumonia.
- Bronchiectasis, although more likely secondary to recurrent infections, bronchiectasis should be considered, as it involves permanent airway damage that predisposes to further infections.

DIAGNOSIS

Foreign body causing recurrent pneumonia

Case study 16

INTRODUCTION

This very pleasant sixty-two-year-old Caucasian man, who smoked ten cigarettes a day for many years, and drank ten pints a week, was married and lived with his wife in their private house. He worked as a public transport bus driver.

SYMPTOMS

The patient was admitted as an emergency where I used to work in north Wales in 1979, complaining about severe numbness in both hands and to a lesser extent in his feet, with muscle cramps in both calves.

In fact the numbness had been happening for the last few weeks, and getting worse with cramps. Had diarrhoea on and off, which did not bother him much, no vomiting, no blood in his motion was noticed. No weight loss, appetite well maintained. No other symptoms.

In the past, he had had a peptic ulcer which failed to respond to medical treatment. Eventually he had a stomach operation, during which, he was told, the surgeon took part of the stomach away.

He suffered from mild asthma, using salbutamol on and off, and was allergic to shellfish, peanuts and eggs. He was not taking any regular medication.

EXAMINATION

This patient was mentally alert, his demeanour good, hydrated, not anaemic clinically, no cyanosis.

Pulse 88/SR, temperature 37^{0}C, BP 145/77

JVP normal, no abnormal finding in the heart or respiratory system.

Upper limbs were symmetrical in shape and length, no muscle wasting, power normal, sensations, all modality normal, tendon reflexes all normal. Lower limbs were also symmetrical in shape and length, no muscle wasting, ulceration, sensation all normal, peripheral pulse was palpable, reflexes normal. Joints full movement and good power.

Abdominal examination, no swelling, old epigastric scar, the rest of the examination was normal. Cranial nerves all normal.

What was most likely diagnosis?

DIFFERENTIAL DIAGNOSIS.

THREE POSSIBLE DIAGNOSES PRESENT THEMSELVES:

- Peripheral neuropathy. However, sensation and reflexes were all normal, no muscle wasting, power was good. So, neuropathy is very unlikely.
- Peripheral vascular disease: this is again unlikely, as the peripheral pulses were all present, with no ulceration.
- Hypocalcaemia remains a possibility, since it causes numbness and cramps. Two tests could be conducted to confirm the diagnosis of hypocalcaemia. Trousseau's sign, in which inflation of a BP machine above systolic pressure induces carpopedal spasm. And Chvostek's sign, by tapping the facial nerve/parotid gland in front of the ear, which causes the facial muscles to twitch.
- Blood tests results confirmed hypocalcaemia.
- The patient's peptic ulcer was the principal contributor to

his hypocalcaemia. The patient's peptic ulcer required a stomach operation. Before the invention of histamine H2-receptor antagonists and PPI medication, surgical treatment for peptic ulcer was common practice. And one of the complications of a partial gastrectomy is

- Hypocalcaemia caused by post-cibal (dumping) syndrome.

LESSONS LEARNED

- It is important to be aware of the complication of old surgical treatment for peptic ulcer.
- Checking for Trousseau's and Chvostek's signs will help in diagnosing suspected hypocalcaemia.
- Hypocalcaemia can disable a patient and threaten his or her life.

Case study 17

INTRODUCTION

The patient was a nine-month-old baby boy, his parents' first child, born four weeks premature by normal vaginal delivery. He lived with his parents in a privately-owned house in the suburbs. The baby's immunisations were up to date, and the only other medical issue of note was mild atopic eczema which had been treated with moisturisers.

SYMPTOMS

On Sunday night, his parents noticed a swelling in the right iliac fossa. The child was crying, vomited once, and opened his bowels as normal. The parents gave him paracetamol, and the child became relatively settled. His father contacted the out-of-hours (OOH) centre and booked an appointment for 10 pm. They managed to see the doctor at 11 pm.

After completing the consultation, and discussion with the family, the doctor advised them to contact their GP in the morning. He gave them a copy of the consultation record to take to the GP.

The family contacted the practice and made an urgent appointment. The father handed over the sealed envelope containing the details of the previous night's consultation, in which the OOH doctor describes finding a lump in the right inguinal area, and suggests to the GP that the child should be referred for an ultrasound scan. The child was at this time very unsettled and screaming.

EXAMINATION

I made a rapid examination, as the child was irritable, and there was no point wasting time. The lump was hard and tender. I realised that it was not the bowels or an inguinal hernia.

> What was the likely diagnosis?
> What would be your action plan in this sort of situation?

TREATMENT

The situation was urgent, contacted the on-call paediatric surgeon at the appropriate hospital and explained my urgent concern to him. He the letter ready to check, sign and be given to the parents for the hospital surgeon.

I advised the parents to take the child to hospital and inform the hospital staff that the case was urgent, and the surgeon should be informed immediately (routine triage of such letters can take a bit of time in the emergency department). Every minute was vital in this case.

The surgeon attended immediately, since he had already been informed about the provisional diagnosis as soon as the pre-operative preparation had been completed, the child was taken to theatre.

The operation was completed. Unfortunately, our worst fears were realised. The child's testicle was gangrenous and needed to be removed. It was a shock to the family; as they never expected such a thing to happen to their first child.

Unfortunately a complaint was inevitable; sadly, I believe was hard to defend. The parents asked why this child had to wait until the morning to see the GP and the diagnoses was missed otherwise had to be referred immediately to deal with the problem. Obviously, the parents were very distressed as one of the testicles has been removed and they believed it was a late referral to the hospital.

It was a sad case. It illustrated the importance of being able to distinguish between inguinal hernia, ectopic testicle and renal cyst. I am aware that the diagnosis can sometimes be difficult, but in this case, onset was rapid, the lump was hard and tender, and there was no palpable testicle in the affected side in the scrotum (an under-developed scrotum is big clue to the possibility of an undescended testicle).

If you are unsure, refer to the hospital, no one can be criticised for doing so.

The right testicle alone is affected in 50 per cent of cases; the left alone in 39 per cent of cases, while double arrested descent occurs in 20 per cent of cases.

The testis may be a) retained within the abdomen, extraperitoneal, b) in the inguinal canal, or c) in the superficial sub inguinal pouch, called retractile testis,

Hazards of incomplete descent are as follows:

- Sterile in bilateral cases.
- Torsion.
- Epididymo-orchitis on the right side is difficult to differentiate from acute appendicitis.
- Atrophy, even before puberty.
- The best age for the operation is before one year of age.
- When both testes are impalpable, the condition is called bilateral cryptorchidism.

LESSONS LEARNED

- Testicular torsion is an emergency which may be difficult to differentiate from inguinal hernia.
- In 20 per cent bilateral, examine both sides, and refer to hospital if not sure.
- The best age for operation is before the age of one year.
- Undescended testicle (intra-abdominal) is liable to get malignant.
- Always speak to hospital surgeon involved to avoid delay, could lead to gangrene.

Case study 18

65-year-old Asian lady, originally from India, now living in the UK in a bungalow with her dependent husband. Her husband had suffered a right-sided stroke a few years before. She had never smoked, was a social drinker, and worked for a few years at a DIY store and as a shop assistant before retiring at the age of sixty-four. She had been active, looking after her husband and managing the household well. She typically went to local shops weekly, driving her small Peugeot car.

SYMPTOMS

About twelve months earlier, she noticed her mild asthma was worsening, and salbutamol was no longer helping, despite using it several times a week. She requested a new supply of her salbutamol inhaler, but her asthma progressively worsened week by week. Finally, she found herself unable to cope.

In January, she called for a home visit because she couldn't leave her dependent husband alone, as she was expecting a gas engineer.

After morning surgery, I went to see her. She opened the front door and sat on the settee, struggling to breathe. After a few minutes, she was able to talk to some extent. She mentioned that over the past few weeks, her breathing had become worse. She denied coughing up blood, chest pain, or feeling feverish. She said she was struggling with housework, but her daughter, who lived nearby, was helping as much as possible. She denied coughing up phlegm.

Her past medical history included mild asthma for many years, gout (no recent flares), and well-controlled hypertension.

She was on regular medication: amlodipine 5 mg once daily and allopurinol for her gout. She had no known allergies.

EXAMINATION

The patient was out of breath with intercostal recessions.
Temperature 36.8°C
Oxygen saturation 96%
No obvious central cyanosis
Pulse 110 bpm SR
BP 115/65
Pulsus paradoxus: 5
Trachea central
Bilateral expiratory wheeze, no crepitations
No signs indicating pneumothorax
Heart examination was unremarkable
No swelling in the ankles or signs of DVT

What would be your current action plan?

TREATMENT

After reviewing the NICE guidelines for hospital admission, decided to treat her at home. Retrieved the nebuliser from the car and administered 2.5 ml of nebulised salbutamol. In the meantime, gave her 200 mg of hydrocortisone intravenously, as she had easy veins for IV access. Observing her, she started to improve within a few minutes. After twenty minutes, all observations were reassuring, left her with a prescription for oral steroids (prednisolone 5 mg tablets, starting dose 40 mg, to be tapered off on a sliding scale). Arranged for her to see me at the practice in a week.

When she was reviewed a week later, everything was going well, started her on a steroid inhaler (beclometasone 200 mcg, two puffs twice daily). I checked her inhaler technique, advised her to use salbutamol as needed, and to finish her oral steroids as instructed. I planned to review her again in four weeks.

SUBSEQUENT DEVELOPMENTS

After completing the course of steroids, she experienced another asthma attack. An ambulance was called, and she was taken to the hospital. She was kept overnight and prescribed another course of steroid tablets and amoxicillin for one week. A chest X-ray was performed and was normal, and her blood tests were satisfactory.

Unfortunately, once she finished the steroids, her asthma symptoms returned.

SUBSEQUENT TREATMENT

I upgraded her asthma medication according to NICE guidelines. However, her asthma remained completely uncontrollable without a considerably high dose of steroids.

WHAT WOULD BE YOUR NEXT STEP AT THAT TIME?

case referral. I contacted the hospital's chest clinic for an urgent appointment. The hospital responded positively, and she attended the clinic within a week.

The consultant reviewed my referral letter and requested blood tests and a repeat chest X-ray. All results were normal. She was reassured and advised to continue her upgraded medication regimen. She was discharged back to community care, with a diagnosis of severe asthma. However, we were back to square one, as her symptoms persisted.

DIFFERENTIAL DIAGNOSIS

It was challenging to pinpoint the problem, but several conditions were considered:

- Pulmonary TB: chest X-rays were negative on two occasions, and she had no fever, night sweats, or weight loss.
- Lung cancer: non-smoker, no haemoptysis, clubbing, or weight loss.
- Fungal chest infection: sputum samples were negative.
- Cardiac asthma: this did not fit the clinical picture.
- Compliance, I checked her compliance multiple times, and it was fine.
- We decided to refer her for a CT scan, although we weren't entirely sure what we were looking for. The CT scan provided the breakthrough we needed.

> Could you guess, what might have been the diagnosis was at that time?

RIGHT MIDDLE LOBE BRONCHIECTASIS.

High-resolution computed tomography (HRCT) is the cornerstone for diagnosing bronchiectasis and other chest lesions. It is non-invasive and highly specific.

Findings in bronchiectasis: dilated airways lying adjacent to pulmonary artery branches create a "ring sign."

There is non-uniform bronchial dilatation, and there are clusters of thin-walled cystic spaces.

HOSPITAL ADMISSION INDICATIONS:

- Irregular heart rhythm
- Oxygen saturation less than 92 per cent
- Central cyanosis
- Silent chest
- Hypotension
- Altered consciousness
- Inability to speak
- Exhaustion
- Peak flow less than 33 per cent of best or predicted value
- Poor respiratory effort
- Lessons learned
- Always consider the differential diagnosis of poorly controlled asthma.
- HRCT is crucial in diagnosing chest problems.
- Don't stop investigating when the hospital has reached its "final destination." Keep trying - you may find the answer!
- Bronchiectasis is one of the main causes of poorly controlled asthma.

Case study 19

INTRODUCTION

This seventeen-year-old girl, a happy, well-disciplined second-year sixth form student, had never smoked, was a social drinker, was living with her parents.

PAST MEDICAL HISTORY

She had suffered from asthma since childhood (worse in summer); for this she had a salbutamol inhaler, used PRN. She also had a topic eczema for many years, using over-the-counter moisturisers to treat it. She had an allergy to pollen.

SYMPTOMS

She was booked as an emergency on a cold, busy morning. After ten minutes, the receptionist alerted me that the emergency patient had arrived. I called her in, aiming to stick to practice protocol, ensuring emergency cases are not kept waiting for more than fifteen minutes.

She walked in accompanied by her mother, slightly bending forward, with her hand on her abdomen. This was unusual for her, as she always walked in with a smile and full of confidence. I gave a warm welcome to her and her mother.

She stated she had been experiencing abdominal pain for the past three days, with occasional vomiting but no diarrhoea. The pain was getting worse, mostly in the lower abdomen, slightly to the right side, constant, with no urinary symptoms. She mentioned her periods were regular and expected soon. She was using condoms, and her last sexual intercourse was a week ago.

She said she had never experienced this type of pain before and had not noticed any skin rash.

EXAMINATION

The patient was in considerable pain. hydrated, but with no obvious rash.

Temperature 37.5°C, Pulse 100 bpm SR, BP 119/62, Oxygen saturation 99%

Abdominal examination: No rash or swelling, but tenderness in the lower right abdomen with typical rebound tenderness. The rest of the physical examination was unremarkable

TREATMENT

I requested a urine sample for a dipstick test to rule out a urinary tract infection and for a pregnancy test to ensure it wasn't an ectopic pregnancy. Both tests were negative. At this point, I explained to her mother that it looked like acute appendicitis, and she needed to go to the hospital to be assessed by the surgical team. I reassured her that this is a common medical emergency in her age group. Her mother agreed to take her to the hospital, and I provided a letter for the surgical ward.

Two days later, her mother called the practice to let us know that she had undergone an appendectomy via laparoscopy and was recovering at home.

SUBSEQUENT TREATMENT

Two days after that, her mother called again requesting a home visit, saying her daughter was not feeling well and was in considerable pain. I saw her after morning surgery. She was in pain, tachycardic, and had a tender abdomen. I contacted the surgical department, and she was admitted immediately. Upon reassessment in theatre, they found a pelvic haematoma, evacuated the blood, and sorted out the source of the bleeding. She was sent home two days later.

SUBSEQUENT DEVELOPMENTS AND TREATMENT.

She was doing well for a week, but then the abdominal pain returned, although without vomiting. Her mother promptly took her to A&E, where the surgical team assessed her, reassured her, and sent her home with painkillers.

However, she did not improve and continued to experience pain. Her mother took her to A&E twice more in the following four days, but she was sent home again each time.

and explained everything that had happened recently. She looked very unwell pale, with a temperature of 37.8°C, Pulse 112 bpm SR, BP

100/60 and abdominal discomfort with tenderness

> What do you think went wrong?
> What would be your action plan at that time?

I took blood samples and sent them to the hospital, telling her I would contact her before 6 pm. When I received the blood results, they showed an ESR of 79, WBC of 17,000, and HB of 9.5, with normal renal and liver function tests. I contacted the surgical team, explained the situation, and provided the latest blood test results.

I then requested an immediate ambulance after informing the patient that she needed to attend the surgical ward. She was admitted and assessed upon arrival. Following an MRI scan, she was taken to theatre again for another laparoscopy, where they stated the problem had been resolved.

She was discharged home after seven days and felt much better after a long, difficult journey.

What was likely the diagnosis?

Pelvic abscess, which was evacuated, followed by a course of antibiotics, initially intravenous for two days, then orally for five days.

LESSONS LEARNED

- Patients with frequent attendance need to be taken seriously
- Be aware of possible laparoscopic complications.
- Blood results showing leukocytosis indicate an infectious problem, find the source.
- Clearance from A&E does not mean the end of the story. The GP must continue to dig deeper to find the cause of the problem.

Case study 20

INTRODUCTION

This fifty-eight-year-old man had been registered in the practice with his family since 1998. He had never smoked and drank 10 pints a week. He lived in a semi-detached house with his wife.

PAST MEDICAL HISTORY

In the past, he had suffered from hypertension, well controlled gout, IBS. He had been prescribed allopurinol for his gout, and lisinopril O D for blood pressure. He had a peanut allergy. In 2000, routine blood tests FBC, showed MCV 101(Normal 78 - 98), He suffered from eczema for a long time, used to attend local hospital clinic, was prescribed few creams, but none really worked well. He still had intense itching, now he was just used to it. Otherwise, he was fit and well, with no shortness of breath. I asked again for details of his alcohol consumption, he confirmed maximum ten pints a week. He stated that his diet included fruits and vegetables daily.

SYMPTOMS

The patient complained of intense itching. He had a skin rash on both knees (front), buttocks and lower back, both elbows, dry, looked like papules, scaly, no ulceration or vesicles. There were scratch marks, no redness to support infective process.

EXAMINATION

The patient looked alert and fit, had no shortness of breath, was not anaemic clinically.

Pulse. 88 SR, saturation 98, RR 18 heart, no cardiomegaly

clinically, heart sound, normal, no added sounds.

Chest, normal shape, breathing sound, normal. Abdominal examination, no jaundice clinically, liver and spleen not palpable.

Upper and lower limbs all normal, CNS, grossly normal.

What was the differential diagnosis at that time?

It was a case of severe itching, with MCV 101 l arranged a few blood tests repeat FBC, request serum folate, B12, liver function tests, Gamma GT, renal function and chest X-ray

When the tests results came back, they were all normal including the chest X- ray, only serum folate was 0.5, normal range 2- 20.

I advised the patient, further tests are needed to determine the cause.

What would you have done next at that time?

I needed to find the cause of his folic acid deficiency. His intake was fine; there must be something wrong with the absorption process. I called him again, suggesting we try certain medication called ?????? for his skin problem, with a review in a week's time, and attend a week later. He was pleased—his skin had improved.

What was this medication?

Medication was DAPSONE

Diagnosis; Dermatitis herpetiform

Dramatic response to dapsone is basically diagnostic.

The patient's folic acid was low, though his intake was fine, so obviously the problem lay in its absorption. Severe itching at the site of the lesions is a characteristic feature; symmetrical sites affected. DH patients have a mild gastrointestinal absorptive defect due to gluten enteropathy, as in patients with coeliac disease.

The patient was referred to a local dermatology clinic, where a skin biopsy confirmed diagnosis: he was also referred to a gastroenterologist, endoscopy done and jejunum biopsy confirmed coeliac disease all other blood test arranged for calcium, ferritin.

Malabsorption was the cause of low folate.

DIFFERENTIAL DIAGNOSIS:

Differential diagnosis is wide as many illnesses may cause rash and itching, such as, for example:

- Metabolic disorder, thyroid, diabetes
- Lichen plants
- Pityriasis rosacea
- Lichen simplex chronicus
- Insect bites
- Scabies
- Malignant lymphoma
- Contact dermatitis
- Atopic dermatitis.
- Connective tissue diseases

DIAGNOSIS.

Dermatitis herpetiform

LESSONS LEARNED,

- Diagnosis may be overlooked ln secondary care clinics.
- Finding the cause of the problem is important.
- Never treat symptoms without trying to find the cause of the symptoms

Case study 21

INTRODUCTION

The patient was a thirty-three-year-old Caucasian male, married, with children in secondary school. He was a self-employed accountant, working from home. He was a non-smoker, and consumed alcohol socially.

PAST MEDICAL HISTORY

He was on no regular medication. He had a history of hyperacidity, treated successfully with omeprazole. He had no known allergies.

SYMPTOMS

The patient presented with recurrent episodes of palpitations over the past few months, varying in duration from a few minutes to several hours. He denied experiencing chest pain, blackouts, or neurological symptoms like slurred speech. Notably, there were no signs of sweating, weight loss, or stress and his appetite and sleep patterns remain unaffected.

Frustration was mounting as the patient had sought medical care multiple times without resolution. He had visited A&E on three occasions, consulted his GP twice, and used out-of-hours (OOH) services three times. On each visit, his ECGs and blood tests were reported as normal, leaving him increasingly anxious about the cause of his palpitations.

EXAMINATION

On examination, the patient appeared well, calm, and articulate, with no signs of anaemia or respiratory distress. Vital signs were stable:

Pulse: 88 bpm (sinus rhythm), blood pressure 127/74
Temperature: 37°C
Oxygen saturation: 98%

Cardiac examination revealed normal heart sounds, with no murmurs or signs of heart failure. The chest was clear to auscultation, with normal respiratory expansion, and no abnormalities were detected. Carotid artery examination revealed no bruits, and both upper and lower limb assessments were unremarkable. Neurological findings, including Romberg's test, were normal.

What was the problem, and your action plan?
Although prior assessments indicated no abnormalities.

Recurrent palpitations despite normal investigations raised the suspicion of an arrhythmogenic condition. In this case, WPW syndrome was identified after a meticulous review of the patient's ECG, revealing hallmark features such as a short PR interval and a delta wave (a slurred upstroke of the QRS complex), which had likely been overlooked in prior evaluations. WPW typically affects young, otherwise healthy individuals, and may not be diagnosed unless symptomatic arrhythmias emerge.

WPW Syndrome is a congenital heart condition characterised by the presence of an accessory conduction pathway, the bundle of Kent, which allows electrical impulses to bypass the AV node. This can lead to episodes of supraventricular tachycardia (SVT). Many individuals with WPW remain asymptomatic, but the characteristic ECG changes, such as the delta wave, are present.

When symptomatic, WPW often manifests as palpitations,

dizziness, or even syncope. In rare cases, the syndrome can predispose individuals to more dangerous arrhythmias, including atrial fibrillation, which may escalate to ventricular fibrillation, a life-threatening condition.

To sum up, the characteristics of Wolff-Parkinson-White (WPW) syndrome are:

- Prevalence: WPW is relatively rare but is most frequently seen in younger patients.
- ECG features: short PR interval (<120 ms); delta wave (slurred upstroke of the QRS complex); prolonged QRS complex (>110 ms)
- Symptoms: palpitations, dizziness, and, in rare cases, syncope. WPW can lead to life-threatening arrhythmias.
- Associations: WPW may coexist with congenital cardiac conditions such as mitral valve prolapse and hypertrophic cardiomyopathy.

LESSONS LEARNED

- This case highlights the importance of maintaining a high index of suspicion for conditions like WPW in young patients with recurrent palpitations and repeated normal investigations.
- Missing subtle ECG findings can delay diagnosis and treatment.
- Emergency departments and out-of-hours services, often overwhelmed by patient volume, must exercise vigilance in interpreting ECGs.

- A careful review by specialists can make the difference in diagnosing and managing this potentially serious condition.
- In this case, a timely referral and careful ECG interpretation led to the identification of WPW, allowing for appropriate treatment and follow-up to prevent future complications.

Case study 22

INTRODUCTION

This thirty-seven-year-old man, a self-employed electrician, was a non-smoker, who drank approximately ten pints of alcohol weekly.

He had suffered from recurrent episodes of abdominal pain for several years, previously managed by his GP. He was diagnosed with gallstones following hospital tests and scheduled for elective gallbladder removal. Notably, the patient mentioned jaundice since childhood, which he believed was normal for him and not symptomatic.

There was no family history of jaundice; the patient was married with no children.

PAST MEDICAL HISTORY

The patient had no other significant past medical history, no regular medication, and no known allergies.

EXAMINATION

The patient appeared to be well, not in respiratory distress, and not clinically anaemic.

Vital signs: temperature 36.8°C, pulse 86 bpm regular, BP 146/83 mmHg.

Cardiorespiratory examination: normal chest and heart findings.

Abdominal examination: soft abdomen, no clubbing or spider naevi, no palmar erythema or flapping tremor. Liver not palpable, but spleen enlarged (palpable 3 cm below costal margin)

Neurological examination: grossly normal

DIFFERENTIAL DIAGNOSIS

- Gilbert's syndrome: a benign condition where bilirubin conjugation is mildly impaired, leading to intermittent jaundice.
- Crigler-Najjar syndrome: a more severe form of bilirubin conjugation failure, typically. presenting early in life.
- Dubin-Johnson syndrome: a rare, benign disorder causing chronic jaundice due to impaired hepatic excretion of conjugated bilirubin.
- Rotor syndrome resembles Dubin-Johnson syndrome but lacks liver pigmentation and results from defective bilirubin storage.
- Chronic liver disease: may lead to jaundice and splenomegaly, although other stigmata of liver disease are absent.
- Haemolytic anaemia: conditions like hereditary spherocytosis or sickle cell anaemia can cause chronic jaundice and splenomegaly.
- Excessive alcohol consumption: could contribute to liver dysfunction, though this patient's consumption level does not suggest chronic liver damage.

What was the diagnosis?

Reasons for reaching this conclusion are:

- Lifelong jaundice, the patient's report of being slightly yellow since childhood is a hallmark of hereditary spherocytosis.
- Gallstones, the presence of pigmented gallstones is common in hereditary spherocytosis due to chronic haemolysis.
- Splenomegaly: enlargement of the spleen is frequently associated with this condition.

- Blood film findings, Confirmatory tests would likely reveal spherocytes on the blood smear, which is a key diagnostic feature.

Diagnosis congenital spherocytosis
Characteristics of hereditary spherocytosis are:
Pathophysiology: the condition is characterised by abnormal, spherically shaped red blood cells (spherocytes) that are more prone to destruction by the spleen (hypersplenism).

Clinical presentation: symptoms can range from mild to severe haemolytic anaemia.

Jaundice: episodes of jaundice are common and may have been present since childhood.

Splenomegaly: the spleen is often enlarged, though this is not always the case.

Gallstones: pigmented stones and cholecystitis are frequent presenting symptoms in adulthood.

Blood findings: a blood film would show spherocytes, with a positive family history in 50 per cent of cases. Bilirubin is typically absent in the urine.

Management: splenectomy is highly effective in managing anaemia and symptoms in severe cases, especially where there are recurrent haemolytic crises, family history of the disease, or complications like cholecystitis and cholelithiasis.

LESSONS LEARNED

- In adults with longstanding jaundice and splenomegaly, hereditary spherocytosis should be considered.
- Family history of similar symptoms should be investigated.

- Diagnosis can be confirmed with simple blood tests, including a blood smear for spherocytes.

Case study 23

INTRODUCTION

The patient was a sixty-two-year-old Afro-Caribbean man, a public bus driver for the last twenty years. He had never smoked and drank two pints five times a week. He had never married, had no children and lived alone in a council house. He was active in the local community, attending church on Sundays.

PAST MEDICAL HISTORY

He had hypertension (controlled with amlodipine 5 mg daily) and benign prostatic hypertrophy (on finasteride 5 mg daily). He had no known allergies.

SYMPTOMS

The patient had been feeling unwell for the past four weeks. His symptoms were lethargy, loss of energy, absence from church, poor appetite, nausea, weight loss, upper back pain (wandering, difficult to localise, no rash or radiation), increased urination (polyuria) with no signs of infection or diabetes (normal blood glucose).

The previous week he had experienced severe epigastric pain without radiation and three episodes of vomiting (no blood or coffee-ground appearance). Over-the-counter painkillers and tonics from a health shop were ineffective.

EXAMINATION

Vital signs: BP 138/78 mmHg, pulse 100 bpm, saturation 98%, temperature 36.8°C;
No jaundice, not clinically anaemic, no shortness of breath;

No palpable neck lumps, chest clear, heart sounds normal;
Abdomen: epigastric discomfort but otherwise normal;
Upper thoracic tenderness on palpation, no obvious lumps or other abnormalities in limbs; Neurological examination unremarkable.

TREATMENT (INITIAL)

Prescribed omeprazole for suspected gastrointestinal involvement. Blood tests requested: FBC, ESR, CRP, LFTs, renal function (glucose normal on the spot). The patient was advised to return for a follow-up with results in a week.

However, that weekend, the patient felt worse and went to the hospital. He was hospitalised for three weeks, treated, and felt better upon discharge. He requested a sick note and medication from the hospital discharge letter.

DIAGNOSIS

Multiple myeloma

Multiple myeloma, a malignant plasma cell disorder

Polyuria with normal glucose suggests hypercalcaemia, a common symptom of multiple myeloma.

Upper back pain and tenderness likely due to bone involvement (vertebral compression fractures or lytic lesions).

Weight loss in a non-smoker suggests an underlying malignant process.

Vomiting and epigastric pain could be manifestations of hypercalcaemia or related gastrointestinal disturbances.

The patient's ethnicity is significant because Afro-Caribbean individuals have a threefold higher risk of developing multiple myeloma.

CHARACTERISTICS OF MULTIPLE MYELOMA:

- Bone involvement: Commonly presents with bone pain (often in the back) due to lytic lesions or fractures.
- Renal damage: Light chains produced by malignant plasma cells can lead to kidney dysfunction
- Hypercalcaemia: Often presents with polyuria, nausea, vomiting, and abdominal pain.
- Anaemia: Common due to bone marrow infiltration by malignant cells, leading to fatigue.
- Infection: Myeloma patients are prone to infections like pneumonia, which may cause significant morbidity and mortality.

EPIDEMIOLOGY:

Incidence is approximately 11 cases per 100,000 people.
Peak incidence occurs between the ages of sixty and seventy.
Afro-Caribbean individuals are disproportionately affected.
Multiple myeloma can be asymptomatic for years before diagnosis, with symptoms often arising from bone involvement, renal dysfunction, or infection.

LABORATORY FINDINGS

A very high ESR (erythrocyte sedimentation rate) is characteristic.

- Diagnosis is confirmed by detecting monoclonal paraprotein in the blood or urine and bone marrow biopsy showing abnormal plasma cells.

LESSONS LEARNED

- Multiple myeloma can present with vague, non-specific symptoms such as back pain, weight loss, polyuria, and gastrointestinal issues
- Hypercalcaemia should always be considered in cases of polyuria with normal blood glucose and unexplained gastrointestinal symptoms.
- ESR is critical diagnostic clue, and very high levels should raise suspicion of myeloma or other serious underlying conditions.

Case study 24

INTRODUCTION

In the summer of 1984, during the first week of September, I agreed to cover a morning surgery session for a company supplying medical staff for out-of-hours (OOH) service on a temporary basis. The surgery was in a beautiful, green area, and it was a relatively small practice. Having recently finished my trainee year; I had limited experience in general practice.

The session began at 9 am. After seeing my second patient, one of the receptionists came into the room and informed me that a baby had arrived without an appointment. The parents were concerned and asked if I could see the baby next. Given that it was an infant and the parents were worried, agreed immediately.

When they entered, welcomed them and introduced me. The mother, who took the lead in conveying the information, explained that their baby was five weeks and two days old, born full-term via normal delivery, and breastfed. Up until that point, everything had been going well with their first child. He had been putting on weight and appeared healthy.

The mother told me that the trouble started that morning around 6 am when she noticed the baby vomiting. At first, he vomited several times but then stopped for about 30 minutes. However, after she gave him some boiled water with minimal juice, the vomiting resumed. What worried her the most was that she had noticed coffee-ground vomit in the baby's vomit, which made her panic. They decided to come directly to the surgery for help.

Upon further questioning, the mother denied any prior history of illness, including a runny nose, fever, or cough. The baby had been feeding normally and had even been fed once just before they made their way to the surgery. The baby was not on any medication, and there was no known history of allergies.

EXAMINATION

The baby was alert but appeared slightly uncomfortable.

Vital signs: Stable, but slightly tachycardic (heart rate mildly elevated for age).

Abdomen: Soft, non-tender, no palpable masses or distension.

Mouth: No obvious signs of infection or dehydration (mucous membranes were moist).

Chest: Clear breath sounds bilaterally, no signs of respiratory distress.

Skin: Normal colour, no rashes or bruises noted.

I was concerned by the coffee-ground vomit, which is indicative of upper gastrointestinal bleeding. This finding was worrying to the parents; but l reassured them,

What was likely the diagnosis and your action plan?

TREATMENT

The baby was referred to the hospital for surgery. I contacted the paediatric team at the hospital to provide them with the details and ensure the baby would be seen quickly.

Potential complications could be dehydration, hypokalaemia or metabolic alkalosis.

Diagnosis; congenital pyloric stenosis

LESSONS LEARNED

- Coffee-ground vomit in infants should always be treated as a medical emergency, as it indicates gastrointestinal bleeding.
- In cases where symptoms are subtle, such as the absence of fever or respiratory symptoms,
- It is crucial to listen carefully to parents' concerns and conduct a thorough examination.
- Rapid referral to a hospital is essential in such cases to prevent complications.

Case study 25

INTRODUCTION

The patient was a twenty-six-year-old female, registered in the practice since the age of six, never smoked, drank socially, and worked in the NHS physiotherapy department at a local hospital. She was single, lived with her parents, and was the only child. She described her life as happy and fulfilling.

SYMPTOMS

At the age of twenty-two, she presented with complaints of abdominal pain that had persisted for several months, primarily on the right side of the mid and lower abdomen. She had been managing the pain with over-the-counter painkillers due to her busy schedule. Her menstrual cycle was regular, and the pain was intermittent, lasting for a few days before subsiding. She reported occasional diarrhoea, but no blood was noticed. There were no symptoms of heartburn, and the pain did not radiate to her back. She denied urinary symptoms, weight loss, or a reduction in appetite. Her medical history included only childhood illnesses, and she had no known allergies.

EXAMINATION

The patient appeared well, confident, and was not anaemic clinically. She had no shortness of breath.

Pulse: 84 bpm, sinus rhythm.

Blood pressure: 124/69 mmHg.

Temperature: 36.9°C.

Height: 165 cm.

Weight: 66 kg.
Oxygen saturation: 99%.
No jaundice was noted.
Abdominal examination: Soft, non-tender, no palpable lumps, no organomegaly.
The remainder of the clinical examination was normal.

TREATMENT (INITIAL)

Given the non-specific symptoms and the absence of abnormal physical signs, I reassured her, and we discussed the possibility of irritable bowel syndrome (IBS), which is a common condition. I advised her to take over-the-counter antispasmodics and monitor her symptoms.

FURTHER SYMPTOMS

Two months later, she saw another GP at the practice with the same complaint. She was reassured again, and no further follow-up was planned. However, three months later, she returned to me, reporting that the pain was worsening and interfering with her life. On examination, there were still no new signs.

At this point, I arranged for a series of tests:

Full blood count (FBC); Liver function tests (LFTs);
Renal function tests;
C-reactive protein (CRP);
Erythrocyte sedimentation rate (ESR);
Faecal occult blood test;
Ultrasound of the abdomen and pelvis.

A few days later, the results were reviewed, and all investigations came back normal. The patient was relieved but asked, "What should I do now, Doctor? Would you mind referring me to see someone in the hospital?" Considering her frustration and the impact on her quality of life, I agreed to refer her to a gynaecologist.

Two months later, I received a clinic letter from the hospital. The gynaecologist had found no gynaecological problems and suggested a referral to a gastroenterologist, suspecting IBS. The tone of the letter was somewhat dismissive.

What was the possible diagnosis and your action plan?

Two months after the gastroenterologist referral, I received a letter from a private hospital detailing her consultation, investigation, diagnosis and planned treatment.

DIFFERENTIAL DIAGNOSIS:

The symptoms were vague, leading to a wide range of possible diagnoses:

- Pelvic Inflammatory Disease (PID): Symptoms include fatigue, lethargy, malaise, low-grade fever, pelvic pain, and congestive dysmenorrhoea. However, the patient's pain was in the abdomen, not the pelvis, and there was no dysmenorrhoea.
- Ectopic pregnancy: Not applicable as she was not pregnant, and the history was too long.
- Torsion of an ovarian cyst: This would have been detected on the ultrasound.
- Uterine fibroid: The ultrasound was negative for fibroids.

DIAGNOSIS

Endometriosis of the right ovary with pelvic adhesions.

CHARACTERISTICS OF ENDOMETRIOSIS.

Endometriosis is a chronic oestrogen-dependent condition characterised by the growth of endometrial tissue outside the uterine cavity. The only reliable diagnostic test for endometriosis is laparoscopy.

It takes an average of seven and a half years from the onset of symptoms to the diagnosis of endometriosis.

Endometriosis affects approximately 10 per cent of women of reproductive age.

Clinical presentation varies and may include lethargy, lower back pain, constipation, dyspareunia (painful intercourse), dysmenorrhoea (painful periods) and subfertility.

Examination is often normal, though tenderness, lumps, or bluish haemorrhagic nodules may be found on pelvic examination.

Treatment typically involves suppression of ovarian function for at least six months, reducing symptoms in 80-90 per cent of patients.

Treatment should be tailored to the individual, with surgical options considered in selected cases.

LESSONS LEARNED

Endometriosis has a highly variable clinical presentation, ranging from severe symptoms to no symptoms at all. In women of reproductive age with unexplained abdominal pain, it is important to consider endometriosis, even though it is less common in women under thirty years old.

Case study 26

INTRODUCTION

This sixty-year-old Caucasian male had recently retired after working as a manager at Curry's retail store for twenty years. He had been a smoker, consuming twenty cigarettes a day since the age of eighteen, but stopped smoking on his retirement date. He lived with his wife in a bungalow and did not drink alcohol.

SYMPTOMS

Approximately four weeks prior, he started noticing breathing difficulties. He had long-standing chronic obstructive pulmonary disease (COPD) but was now wheezing at night and had a persistent cough. He denied night sweats, coughing up blood, chest pain, or weight loss. He mentioned attending an ophthalmology clinic a week before the onset of his symptoms and suspected he may have contracted something from the hospital. His eye drops were changed from Seriban to Ganfort as his previous drops were not effective.

PAST MEDICAL HISTORY

The patient had a history of multiple conditions including ischemic heart disease (IHD), high blood pressure (HBP), COPD, and glaucoma. He was allergic to tetracycline and was taking several regular medications, including Atrovent inhaler, Combicort turbohaler, amlodipine tablets, isosorbide mononitrate tablets, and atorvastatin for high cholesterol.

EXAMINATION

Observations following examination of the patient were as follows:

- Pleasant and relaxed
- Audible wheeze, minimal central cyanosis
- Oxygen saturation: 93%
- No flapping tremors
- Pulse: 100 bpm, sinus rhythm
- Temperature: 37.1°C
- Jugular venous pressure (JVP): Normal
- Blood pressure: 134/78 mmHg
- Congested eyes with warm limbs
- Barrel-shaped chest, expansion: 3 cm
- Chest: Few scattered wheezes and crackles on both sides
- Heart: No abnormal signs detected
- Lower limbs: Minimal ankle oedema
- Mentally well, no CNS abnormalities, no signs of DVT

DIAGNOSTIC COMPLEXITY

This is a case of long-standing multi-morbidity with recent deterioration. Potential causes could include

- Poor medication compliance (checked, no issues)
- Poor inhaler technique (checked, no issues)
- Chest infection following the hospital visit (possible, though temperature was normal)
- Small pulmonary embolism (no cough or DVT signs, but the absence of DVT does not rule it out)
- Small pneumothorax (no clinical signs to support this).

TREATMENT (INITIAL)

Suspecting a possible infection, I prescribed a one-week course of amoxicillin and requested an urgent chest X-ray to rule out other possibilities. A week later, the patient returned. The radiology report showed no abnormalities apart from COPD signs. On examination, there were no changes in chest findings.

I then decided to try a course of steroids, explaining the situation to the patient, who agreed. A week later, he returned with only partial improvement, with persistent wheezing.

FURTHER TREATMENT

I felt I needed help at this stage, so I contacted the chest clinic, where the patient was booked for an appointment. A week later, the patient returned with handwritten notes from the chest clinic, suggesting a new treatment regimen. I followed the consultant's recommendations and scheduled a review for a week later. At the follow-up, the patient said, "I'm fine now, and thank you for referring me to the hospital."

What was the diagnosis?

Drug-induced problem

Drug-induced issues are common in general practice. Upon reflecting on the patient's history, the clue was in his statement that the symptoms started after his hospital visit, during which his eye drops were changed. He was initially using Seriban (a prostaglandin analogue, bimatoprost) and it was changed to Ganfort (bimatoprost combined with timolol). Timolol, a beta-blocker, is contraindicated in patients with asthma and COPD due to its potential to exacerbate respiratory symptoms, even though it is administered as eye drops.

LESSONS LEARNED

- Listening carefully to the patient is crucial.
- Even eye drops can be absorbed systemically and cause adverse effects.
- The clinic may have overlooked the patient's history of COPD.
- When brand names are used, it's important to check the generic components to fully understand the treatment and its potential interactions.

Case study 27

INTRODUCTION

The patient was a sixth-eight-year-old Afro-Caribbean male, who moved to the UK in 1969, worked for Rover Cars in midlands for twenty years before retiring at the age of sixty-five. He never smoked and drank two pints of beer every night. His wife had died a few years before, and he was now living alone in private accommodation. He described his life as content, socialising with his Afro-Caribbean community.

PAST MEDICAL HISTORY

He had a history of high blood pressure for three years, for which he was taking amlodipine. He was not allergic to any known agents.

SYMPTOMS

His health had been good until four weeks prior to his attendance at the out-of-hours (OOH) clinic where I saw him. Initially, he felt weak and lacking energy, but there were no other symptoms. He waited a week before deciding to see his GP, who did not find anything wrong and reassured him.

Despite this, his symptoms did not improve. He then developed indigestion but denied any vomiting or diarrhoea. He tried over-the-counter antacids without relief. He decided to visit A&E, where he was examined and given antacids for upper abdominal pain. He was advised to see his GP if further treatment was needed.

The following day, dissatisfied with the hospital visit, he returned to his GP, who started him on omeprazole (PPI). Three days later, his symptoms worsened. He contacted the GP practice again, requesting to see the doctor, but the receptionist informed him that the GP was busy and would call after surgery. He waited for the call until 10 pm, but the GP did not call. Frustrated, he attended the OOH clinic, where I saw him.

He explained that he had no diarrhoea or vomiting, only persistent indigestion without radiation. His neighbour accompanied him to the appointment.

EXAMINATION,

Observations following examination of the patient were as follows:

- Pleasant, no shortness of breath
- Not clinically anaemic
- Temperature: 36.6°C
- Pulse: 100 bpm, sinus rhythm
- Blood pressure: 114/64 mmHg
- Oxygen saturation: 97%
- Abdomen: No tenderness, lumps, or organomegaly
- Chest and heart: Unremarkable
- No ankle oedema or jaundice

I couldn't find anything particularly concerning at that point. I decided to give him a prescription alongside his omeprazole and printed out a prescription for tablets and handed it to him. As he stood up to leave, he suddenly mentioned, "Doc, I've lost so much weight." Immediately, I asked him to hand back the prescription and sit down again.

> What was the reason, I asked him to sit down?

It only took me two minutes to reach an accurate diagnosis:

SUBSEQUENT TREATMENT

I checked his blood glucose level, which was extremely high—so high that it was outside the reading capacity of the machine. I contacted the hospital immediately and arranged for his admission.

Diagnosis; diabetic keto acidosis

This case illustrates the different ways in which diabetes mellitus can present itself:

- Incidental findings of high blood sugar, for example during preoperative checks or eye examinations.
- Classical symptoms such as polyuria, polydipsia, and weight loss.
- Skin infections, such as balanitis.
- Atypical presentations, particularly in adults, were indigestion, as in this case, can be the primary concern.

LESSONS LEARNED

- Multiple attendances for the same issue should always be taken seriously.
- The last patient of the clinic or OOH session can be at risk of misdiagnosis because of the tendency to rush due to time constraints. It's essential to remain thorough and vigilant.
- A thorough medical history is crucial to minimising avoidable mistakes.
- Diabetic ketoacidosis is fatal if not identified and treated promptly.
- Indigestion as a symptom of DKA can be misleading, especially in older adults.

Case study 28

INTRODUCTION

This thirty-five-year-old Caucasian female, single, living with her parents in a council flat on the fifth floor, had worked for an accounting firm for the last fifteen years. She joined our practice at the age of fifteen, along with her family. She had never smoked and drank socially with friends about once a week.

SYMPTOMS

She had been healthy until three months before when she started feeling tired, with general aches and pains, and joint aches. She denied any joint swelling or morning stiffness. Eight weeks ago, she visited the practice after trying over-the-counter painkillers with minimal relief.

PAST MEDICAL HISTORY

Her past medical history included atopic dermatitis during childhood, which had since cleared. She was not currently on any medication for it and denied any known allergies or regular medications.

EXAMINATION

Upon examination, she did not appear as her usual lively and happy self. She was not clinically anaemic, and her respiratory rate was 18. Her pulse was 100 bpm (sinus rhythm), her temperature was 37°C, and there were no skin rashes or marks. Chest expansion and breath sounds were satisfactory, with no abnormal findings. Her blood pressure was recorded at 110/74, and her oxygen saturation was 98%. Heart sounds were normal with no evidence of cardiomegaly. Mentally, there were no signs of active psychosis; she only seemed down, which could be explained by feeling unwell.

Her limbs were symmetrical in shape and length, with no joint deformities and full range of movement. Her lower limbs also showed no obvious abnormalities, and her reflexes were normal. Neck and throat examinations were normal, and her abdominal examination revealed no issues.

I had a long discussion with her, explaining that her symptoms could be due to a viral illness, given the lack of significant findings on examination. I suggested she take two weeks off work and return for a follow-up appointment. She accepted this plan.

FURTHER SYMPTOMS

She returned to the practice with her mother, stating that she felt no better and was getting worse. I examined her again but found no new signs.

FURTHER TREATMENT

Requested several blood tests, including FBC, ESR, LFTs, rheumatoid factor, ANA, complement levels, and U&E. I gave her the form to attend the phlebotomy department at the local hospital the following morning. She was advised to book an appointment in one week for a review, expecting the blood test results to be available by then.

A week later, she attended her appointment with her mother again, understandably concerned. reviewed her blood test results, which showed:

- CRP: 78
- ESR: 90

The rest of the blood tests were satisfactory.

Contacted the rheumatologist at the local hospital to discuss the case and determine the best course of action. The rheumatologist kindly agreed to see her in his clinic the following day. Provided her with all the relevant blood test results. Both the patient and her mother were happy with this plan. In the meantime, advised her to remain off work for a further period.

The consultant rheumatologist contacted the practice the next day, suggesting that we start her on anti-inflammatory medication. He mentioned that he was unsure of the exact diagnosis but was investigating further. He promised to keep the practice informed, issued a prescription for naproxen 500 mg twice daily, along with omeprazole 20 mg once daily, adhering to NICE guidelines.

Two weeks later, the patient came in to request more medication. I happened to be standing in the reception area and asked if she could spare a moment to speak with me. She confirmed and asked about her status regarding the medication. She reported that it had helped, but her symptoms kept returning.

It took several more weeks of full investigations by the consultant before a diagnosis was confirmed, and treatment was initiated.

What was the diagnosis?

DIAGNOSIS

Vasculitis

Vasculitis is not an uncommon condition, with approximately

14,000 new cases per year. The causes include:

- Idiopathic (50 per cent)
- Infective (e.g., septic or Henoch-Schönlein purpura, 10-15 per cent)
- Inflammatory disorders (e.g., rheumatoid arthritis, systemic lupus erythematosus, Crohn's disease, 10-15 per cent)
- Neoplastic (less than 5 per cent)
- Vasculitis is a challenging condition to diagnose and is unfortunately not a pleasant one to have. Treatment is usually steroid based. It tends to affect small and medium-sized arteries. Small vessel vasculitis may affect terminal digital arteries, causing nail fold infarcts, leg ulcers or purpura. It can also cause mononeuritis multiplex by occluding the vasa nervorum. Large vessel vasculitis may lead to occlusion of cerebral, coronary, mesenteric, and renal arteries, resulting in catastrophic outcomes such as stroke, heart attack, or intestinal ischemia.

LESSONS LEARNED

- Very high ESR and CRP levels should prompt consideration of connective tissue disorders, vasculitis, or cancers.
- Early referral is crucial to avoid preventable mistakes.
- Vasculitis can present with heart attacks, strokes or skin ulcers.

Case study 29

INTRODUCTION

This seventy-six-year-old retired Polish man worked as a construction engineer and was now living alone after losing his wife a few years ago. He had been a smoker since the age of eighteen, smoking one pack a day, and drank two pints of beer every night. He did not go out much but mingled with a few friends from his own community.

PAST MEDICAL HISTORY

He had hypertension, controlled with water tablets, and gout, controlled with allopurinol for many years. He had no known allergies.

SYMPTOMS

I first saw this patient in 1984, during my second six-month trainee year in general practice. He complained of a headache for the previous few months, affecting only the right temporal area, sometimes extending to the back of his head. No vomiting or additional symptoms were noted. He had been using paracetamol without much relief, and his symptoms worsened. He attended the local hospital emergency department, where they assessed him, conducted basic blood tests including an ESR (which was 12), reassured him, and advised him to continue using paracetamol.

Two months later, he visited the GP practice and saw one of the partners, who requested more blood tests, including another ESR. When reviewed a week later, the results showed no abnormalities, with the ESR now at 10. The GP reassured him that there were no serious problems and prescribed naproxen, an anti-inflammatory, to try.

A month later, he came to the practice again, and I saw him. Reviewed his records, blood tests and previous examinations, all of which were reassuring. He mentioned that he had begun experiencing aches and pains, particularly in his joints, although he denied stiffness and visual disturbances. However, he also noted that he had lost half a stone in weight.

EXAMINATION

Observations following examination of the patient were as follows:

- Clinically, he was not anaemic, jaundiced, or cyanotic.
- Weight: 80 kg
- Height: 179 cm
- Temperature: 37°C
- Pulse: 90 bpm, sinus rhythm
- Blood Pressure: 150/95
- Heart: No abnormalities detected
- No ankle swelling
- Right carotid artery bruit: moderate
- Ankle pulses: palpable
- Temporal arteries: not palpable on both sides
- Chest: Normal shape, with a few scattered wheezes (expected given his long-standing smoking history)

What would be your action plan?

Decided to repeat the blood tests, including the ESR. Arranged for the blood tests to be reviewed in a week. When the patient returned, reviewed the results: full blood count (FBC), renal function, and liver function tests (LFTs) were all normal, but the rheumatoid factor was positive. Despite the reassuring tests, the patient was still suffering from headaches and losing weight. He also reported that both his shoulders and upper arms were painful. Decided to request a C-reactive protein (CRP) test and see him again in a few days.

The blood results came back, and I was surprised to find that his CRP was elevated at 50, despite his ESR remaining normal.

What was the diagnosis? And what treatment would you consider?

Answer:
Contacted the local hospital's rheumatologist to discuss the case and seek advice.

The rheumatologist advised me to start the patient immediately on a steroid, with a starting dose of 40 mg.

Two days later, the patient phoned the practice and stated that he was feeling much better. He confirmed that he would attend his follow-up appointment in three weeks as scheduled.

DIAGNOSTIC COMPLEXITY

This case was a challenge. The patient's symptoms were suggestive of temporal arteritis, with a temporal headache that extended to the occipital area, weight loss, and joint pain. Despite these classic signs, his ESR was normal. However, the patient was getting worse, and his CRP was elevated, indicating an active inflammatory process. The rheumatologist advised against a temporal artery biopsy, as the patient's temporal arteries were not palpable. The risk of the patient losing his sight was high, and I considered that I might end up in the witness box if things went wrong. It was important to focus on treating the patient and his symptoms rather than relying solely on investigations. Temporal arteritis can affect small and medium-sized arteries and may lead to stroke, blindness or heart attacks if left untreated.

The rheumatologist advised against a temporal artery biopsy for two reasons:

- The biopsy results could take a few days which would be too late in an urgent case like this.
- Temporal artery biopsy can sometimes be negative, even in confirmed cases of temporal arteritis. A temporal artery biopsy be negative in about 15 per cent of cases due to: a) Skip lesions – areas of the artery that are unaffected by the disease. b) Inadequate specimen – the biopsy may not capture the affected segment.

LESSONS LEARNED

- CRP can be high while ESR remains normal.
- ESR may be normal in cases of temporal arteritis.
- Temporal artery biopsy may be negative due to the segmental nature of the disease.
- Treat the patient based on clinical signs, serological findings, and response to steroids rather than relying solely on tests.

Case study 30

INTRODUCTION

An eighteen-month-old child, whose single mother was from Romania and did not speak English, was brought to the out-of-hours (OOH) clinic by her friend, who speaks good English. I was working an OOH shift, and our office was in the Accident and Emergency (A&E) department. It was a wet, cold night when the mother brought the child to be seen.

SYMPTOMS

The triage nurse in A&E assessed the child, who had been suffering from a high temperature for the last twenty-four hours and referred him to the OOH triage nurse. After the OOH triage nurse assessed him, the child was referred to an OOH clinician and booked as a routine appointment. The mother and her friend waited to be called.

That night, the OOH clinic was relatively quiet due to the harsh weather, as people tend to stay indoors. After twenty minutes, I called the child and the mother, and her friend sat down. The child was in his mother's lap, looking around with his lovely brown eyes and no visible photophobia.

Introduced myself and asked what the problem was. The mother's friend translated, explaining that the child had had a fever for the last day but no runny nose, cough, or vomiting. At this point, noticed a purpuric rash on the child's cheeks, upper chest and forearms. Asked how long the rash had been present, and the mother confirmed it had been there for a few hours. Wearing gloves, Examined the rash, which was non-blanching rash, and the skin was smooth, ruling out eczema or a local skin infection

TREATMENT

Urgently called the nurse and requested her to take the child to the A&E department immediately and inform the doctor in charge, as suspected meningococcal meningitis, which required swift action. The entire consultation took only a couple of minutes, from the moment the child entered the consulting room to when I asked the nurse to transfer him to the emergency department, which was just twenty metres away.

Two hours later, before the end of my shift, went to the emergency department to inquire about the child. I was informed that the child had crashed, and his blood sugar was 1.5. He was transferred immediately to a highly specialised centre. It was 11 pm. Three days later, followed up again with the emergency department and received the sad news that the child had died at 2.30 am, three hours after his transfer.

Further inquiry revealed that there was a twenty-minute delay in seeing the child at the emergency department. I have no further information regarding the findings and reasons behind the delay. However, I believe a few issues were identified, and measures were put in place to prevent such delays from happening again. The department responded positively to the findings.

The sequence of events involved the child being assessed by triage nurses in the emergency department. They believed it was a case for OOH, and the child was referred to the OOH triage nurse, assessed again, and passed to OOH clinicians for a routine appointment, meaning the child was to be seen within four to six hours.

Two problems can be identified:

- Clinical issues in the initial assessment of the child.
- Communication failure, leading to delays, which possibly affected the outcome.
- Meningococcal meningitis is caused by Neisseria meningitidis and spreads via airborne routes, often in cramped living conditions or during dry, hot weather.

The different presentations of meningitis are:

- Fulminant form: Abrupt onset with shock, widespread purpuric rash, and death within hours.
- Meningitis form: More common, starting with an upper respiratory tract infection for one or two days, followed by classical symptoms and signs of meningitis.
- Chronic meningococcaemia: rare form, with patients feeling unwell for weeks or months, presenting with recurrent fever, sweating, joint pain, and transient rash.
- In children, especially infants, the presentation may differ. Symptoms may include vomiting, irritability, high-pitched crying, and convulsions. In older children, neck stiffness is a late feature and is rarely seen in infants. A bulging fontanelle is a valuable sign in children under eighteen months.
- Meningism (neck stiffness with normal cerebrospinal fluid) can pose a diagnostic challenge, as it may be caused by other conditions such as tonsillitis, otitis media, pyelonephritis, and pneumonia.

LESSONS LEARNED

- Classical symptoms may be absent in children Neck stiffness is a late sign in children

- Clinical suspicion of meningitis requires immediate action—there is no time for prolonged examinations, as time is crucial and greatly affects the outcome
- An efficient triage service is essential.

Case study 31

INTRODUCTION

A fifty-two-year-old lady from Zimbabwe, living in the UK for fifteen years, had recently registered at our practice. She was divorced, lived alone, had a grown-up son, and worked as a community carer. She was a non-smoker, did not consume alcohol, and had no significant past medical history, except for an allergy to penicillin. There were no regular medications in her current routine.

SYMPTOMS

At her initial check-up, the patient appeared well-spoken, happy and asymptomatic, with no shortness of breath or signs of anaemia.

EXAMINATION

Physical examination was largely unremarkable:

- Height: 162 cm
- Weight: 78 kg
- Blood pressure (BP) measured at three intervals: 179/99, 175/100, and 165/97
- Pulse: 80 bpm, regular
- Oxygen saturation: 99%
- Normal heart and lung sounds, no abnormalities in her limbs or central nervous system (CNS)

Given the elevated BP readings, we engaged in a thorough discussion regarding hypertension. I ordered relevant blood tests, including lipid profile, urea and electrolytes, full blood count

(FBC), and HbA1c, all of which returned normal. A follow-up visit was scheduled for a week later.

During her next appointment, the lowest BP reading was still elevated at 164/96.

TREATMENT (INITIAL)

Given the patient's preference for non-pharmaceutical management, we agreed to trial lifestyle modifications. A diet sheet and exercise regimen (150 minutes of moderate exercise per week) were provided, with a review set for four months later.

Unfortunately, despite her efforts, at the four-month review, her BP remained high, and there was no weight change. After a further discussion, she reluctantly agreed to begin antihypertensive medication. As she is of African descent, I initiated treatment with a calcium channel blocker, amlodipine 5 mg, following local guidelines.

A week later, her BP had improved to 140/78. Three weeks after that, it reduced further to 136/76, indicating successful control with amlodipine. She was advised to continue and attend regular reviews.

For the next four years, she attended appointments regularly, but recently, her BP readings began creeping above the recommended levels. Despite her claims of adherence, her BP continued to rise even after increasing the amlodipine dosage and adding further medications per protocol.

At its peak, her BP reached 188/110, with no signs of organ damage or renal abnormalities. All relevant blood work, including renal function and cortisol levels, were normal, ruling out secondary causes like Conn's disease. After maxing out her medication regimen without success, I reached the referral threshold and referred her to a secondary care hypertension clinic.

SUBSEQUENT TREATMENT

The hypertension clinic discontinued her prior medications and prescribed a combination of amlodipine 5 mg and Bendroflumethiazide 2.5 mg. Remarkably, within a month, her BP was well controlled, and she was discharged back to our care.

What was the diagnosis?

Diagnosis; poor compliance

Upon further inquiry, she admitted to the consultant that she had not been taking her medication consistently throughout the treatment process.

LESSONS LEARNED

- Poor compliance is a common but often overlooked cause of uncontrolled chronic conditions, such as hypertension, diabetes, and asthma. Always be vigilant for this possibility when treatment outcomes seem disproportionate to the medical intervention.
- Follow NICE guidelines for the management of hypertension to ensure evidence-based care and timely intervention.
- Refer to secondary care once the treatment threshold is reached or when it becomes apparent that the patient might benefit from a second opinion.

- Patient trust and openness are critical to effective treatment. Early identification of non-compliance can prevent prolonged, unproductive battles with a seemingly resistant condition.
- This case highlights the importance of patient compliance in managing chronic conditions and underscores the need for thorough, open discussions to build trust.

Case study 32

INTRODUCTION

This thirty-one-year-old Polish woman, with reasonable English, was married with children, living in rented accommodation in a Birmingham suburb. She had worked in a meat factory for the past three years. She never smoked, drank occasionally, and lived an active life.

SYMPTOMS

She was perfectly well until one month prior to her first attendance at the practice. She had had intermittent abdominal pain during that month, coming and going, in the central part, no radiation, no symptoms to suggest urinary infection. She had no diarrhoea or constipation, and her periods were regular (her partner used a condom).

She stated that her pain was getting worse, interrupting her sleep, making her feel tired most of the time, struggling to work and look after her family. There was no change in her, appetite and weight. She had had an under-active thyroid for a few years. She had no allergies. She was taking levothyroxine 25 mg o d.

EXAMINATION

Observations following examination of the patient were as follows:
Alert and well, no shortness of breath, not anaemic, no jaundice visible, no rash or bruises, weight 64 kg
Temp 37⁰C, saturation 99, RR 18 .
Respiratory system:, trachea central, expansion normal, breathing sounds normal both sides, no added sounds.

CVS: Pulse 80 , SR, BP 125/67 JVP 2 cm, heart not enlarged clinically, heart sounds normal, no added sounds, no ankle oedema.
Abdomen: No obvious lumps, no bruises, no tenderness or signs of ascites, no bowel sounds detected, no hernia visible or palpable. No organomegaly.
No abnormality in lower and upper limbs.

Central nervous system: Gross examination normal.
Management: (initial)

Arranged blood tests: FBC, LFTS, faecal occult blood, CRP, ESR, urine examination, ultrasound of abdomen and pelvis. The blood test results came through, all normal, but were still waiting for the ultrasound appointment.

The patient had attended A&E twice with abdominal pain but was discharged with pain killers. Her blood tests were all normal.

She then visited the practice and requested referral to hospital. l decided to refer her to the gynaecology clinic. During this time, she attended her ultrasound appointment After attending two appointments, she was discharged by the consultant, as there were no gynaecological problems. No abnormality was detected in the ultrasound scan.

> What would you do next at that time?

FURTHER TREATMENT

The patient was still in pain, so I decided to do a further screening test to include calcium. When two days later the results came back, was surprised to see that calcium levels were considerably high. Requested a parathyroid hormone test; result was high, with low phosphate.

The patient was referred to the endocrinologist to sort things out.

Decided to request an abdominal plane X-ray. I thought it was pointless to request further ultrasound scan as she had had one recently. Contacted the hospital radiology department for the X-ray report, which was e-mailed to the practice. It was a Stag-Horne right kidney stone. Though previous ultrasound scan report was reported normal.

The patient was called and informed of the result of her recent X-ray. She was referred to the urologist.

DIFFERENTIAL DIAGNOSIS

Gall bladder
Kidney stones
Endometriosis
Crohn's disease
TB bowels
Ovarian cancer
Fibroid

DIAGNOSIS

After few months, it was found that she had adenoma of the parathyroid. This was removed by surgery. The urologist dealt with her kidney stone, and the patient was back to normal again.

LESSONS LEARNED

- Always take patient complaints seriously.
- Repeat investigation if you are not convinced, believe patient rather than the - investigation machine. Multiple attendances should raise concern.
- Renal stone may vary in its presentation.
- Hypercalcaemia may cause peptic ulcer. Check calcium in abdominal pain.
- best to detect renal stones is plain x ray or CT.

Case study 33

INTRODUCTION

In the winter of 1987, I was working the night shift in the Midlands, covering an out-of-hours (OOH) service for a group of local practices. The weather was particularly harsh, with heavy snow blanketing the streets, making the already demanding job even more challenging. On this night, I was assigned five routine calls - patients who needed to be seen within six hours. As was my usual approach, I planned to visit the patients in a geographically efficient manner to make the most of my time.

I arrived at my first stop around 7.40 pm. The driveway was completely blocked by a snowdrift, but fortunately, my navigator and I were prepared. Equipped with wellington boots and a sturdy digging spade, we managed to clear a path to the front door. The patient's wife welcomed us into their home, where I found a fifty-one-year-old man lying on the sofa, looking visibly apprehensive. He was a non-smoker, a social drinker, and worked at the Rover car plant in Longbridge.

SYMPTOMS

The patient explained that after finishing his salmon dinner, he suddenly experienced severe pain on the right side of his abdomen. The pain radiated to his back and lasted for about thirty minutes. There had been no vomiting or diarrhoea, and his last bowel movement eighteen hours prior had been normal. Although the pain had subsided somewhat after he applied a hot water bottle, he still appeared anxious. He had taken two paracetamol about an hour before I arrived, which seemed to ease the pain slightly.

EXAMINATION

On examination, the patient was alert but anxious. His pulse was 100 beats per minute, regular, and his blood pressure was elevated at 155/92. He was not sweating, and there was no shortness of breath. His temperature was 36.8°C, and there were no abnormalities found in his heart or chest. The abdominal examination revealed tenderness in the middle third of the right side, but no rebound tenderness or visible bruising.

DIFFERENTIAL DIAGNOSIS

- Gallbladder disease, though possible, the absence of upper-right quadrant pain and jaundice made it less likely.
- Appendicitis, the location and presentation were atypical, though it couldn't be ruled out entirely.
- Crohn's disease or Ulcerative colitis, the lack of bowel changes or bloody diarrhoea made these less likely, though Crohn's can present variably, particularly with involvement at the ilecaecal junction.
- Diverticulitis, Possible, but the presentation wasn't classic.
- Renal stone or infection, certainly within the realm of possibility, given the radiating pain.
- Dissecting aortic aneurysm, although less common, this was a life-threatening condition that required immediate consideration.
- Other causes, Peptic ulcers, pancreatitis, and even colon cancer could not be entirely ruled out.
- Despite the broad differential, one condition stood out in my mind: a dissecting aneurysm of the descending aorta. Given the radiating abdominal pain and the patient's profuse sweating during the episode, this seemed a strong possibility.

TREATMENT

I contacted the local hospital to arrange for the patient to be seen, but the senior registrar on call informed me that they had no available beds. Other hospitals in the area were also unable to accept the patient due to capacity issues.

With the hospital refusing admission, I was left with a critical decision. I firmly explained to the senior registrar that suspected the patient had a potentially life-threatening condition - a dissecting aneurysm - and that no other facility could handle the case. Despite the initial pushback, I insisted that the patient be admitted and sent him to Accident and Emergency (A&E).

At 2 am, followed up with the hospital. The senior registrar had just come out of the theatre and admitted that my diagnosis was accurate - a dissecting aneurysm of the descending aorta. The patient had been taken to theatre in time, and the life-threatening condition was managed successfully.

LESSONS LEARNED

- OOH work can be unpredictable and challenging, especially in adverse weather conditions. The combination of harsh weather, blocked roads and resource limitations made this case particularly difficult.
- Aortic dissection is a rare but critical diagnosis in acute abdominal presentations. It should always be considered, even when the symptoms are not immediately typical.
- Hospitals cannot refuse to treat patients based on bed availability, especially in life-threatening situations.
- As a GP, you must advocate for your patients, even in the face of resistance. It's our duty to ensure that patients

receive the care they need, no matter the circumstances.

- This case serves as a reminder that, in the field of medicine, you often need to trust your instincts and advocate strongly for your patients. Had I not persisted, the outcome for this patient could have been very different. In challenging situations, both clinical skill and determination are essential tools in ensuring the best possible outcome for those in our care

DIAGNOSIS

Dissecting aneurysm.

Case study 34

INTRODUCTION

The patient was an eighty-four-year-old man, widowed for fifteen years, living alone in a council house. He had stopped smoking twelve years previously and did not consume alcohol. Despite his age, he remained relatively independent, managing his own shopping and laundry, and walking his dog daily. His only family support came from his son-in-law, who visited occasionally. His history included thirty years of service in the military, which was relevant when considering his overall health and potential for respiratory exposure during service.

PAST MEDICAL HISTORY

For many years, he had been treated for gout and hypertension, with his current medications being allopurinol (300 mg OD) and amlodipine (5 mg OD). He had no significant allergies.

SYMPTOMS

Two months ago, his health began to decline. His appetite waned, and he developed a persistent cough. Initially, his GP prescribed a course of antibiotics, which proved ineffective. He sought additional relief from over-the-counter cough linctus, but there was no improvement. After four weeks of deteriorating symptoms, including weight loss, worsening cough, shortness of breath, and difficulty sleeping, he changed his GP and registered at a new practice.

EXAMINATION

On physical examination, the patient appeared frail with significant shortness of breath and cyanosis. His weight loss was apparent, and there were minor bruises on his arms, though these could be age-related. He was alert, co-operative, and maintained a good demeanour.

Observations following examination of the patient were as follows:

Respiratory examination

- RR: 24
- No clubbing or cervical lymphadenopathy
- Left lung: normal breath sounds
- Right lung: mid-zone coarse crepitations with expiratory wheeze

Cardiovascular findings

Irregular pulse (88 bpm)

- JVP: 2.5 cm (normal)
- Oxygen saturation: 94%
- BP: 110/70
- No abnormal heart sounds
- Slight ankle swelling with palpable peripheral pulses

Abdominal examination was unremarkable, with no organomegaly.

TREATMENT

Given the patient's significant shortness of breath, frailty, and unilateral chest signs, I made the decision to admit him to the hospital. The possibility of a serious underlying condition, such as lung cancer, was a concern, and a hospital environment was necessary for further investigation and accurate diagnosis. After discussing the case with the medical on-call team, the patient was admitted.

The next morning, the patient's son-in-law returned with the hospital discharge letter. To my surprise, the letter indicated a normal chest X-ray and a recommendation for an outpatient follow-up in six weeks. The renal function was noted to be suboptimal, but no significant respiratory findings were mentioned.

SUBSEQUENT TREATMENT

Despite this, the patient continued to deteriorate. He requested antibiotics, and I, feeling frustrated and questioning the adequacy of the hospital's investigation, prescribed a course of cefalexin (500mg TDS). One week later, his condition worsened, with persistent chest signs and no clinical improvement.

What would you do at this stage?
What do you think went wrong?

Contacted the hospital again, expressing my growing concerns, and the patient was re-admitted. Sadly, his condition rapidly declined. His son-in-law informed me that the hospital had diagnosed lung cancer, and within a few days, the patient passed away.

In the light of the patient's tragic outcome, took immediate steps to address the situation. Contacted the hospital's radiology department and the A&E team to confirm that no chest X-ray had been performed during his recent admission, despite the discharge letter's statement. Further inquiry revealed that the patient's last chest X-ray had been conducted fifteen years ago.

Escalated the matter to the hospital's medical director, who acknowledged that errors had occurred. We held a formal meeting in which I received a sincere apology, and the hospital promised to investigate to ensure such oversights would not be repeated in the future.

LESSONS LEARNED

- Responsibility of vigilance: Even when patients are under the care of a hospital, it is essential for GPs to remain vigilant. If something does not seem right, further inquiry is crucial, as hospitals, like any other medical institution, can make mistakes.
- Pursuing accountability: When a significant error occurs, it is essential to take the issue further to ensure that systemic changes are made to prevent similar incidents in the future.
- Professionalism in adverse outcomes: It is important not to exploit a patient's situation by encouraging complaints or trying to position oneself as a hero.
- Professionalism requires humility, responsibility and a focus on improving patient care.
- This case serves as a reminder that while clinical errors may happen, it is our duty to advocate for our patients and work towards improving the systems in place to prevent harm in the future.

Case study 35

INTRODUCTION

A fifty-three-year-old Asian woman, unable to speak English, had arrived in the UK a few years ago and was living with her family in a multicultural suburb of the city. She had never worked in the UK, and her partner was employed part-time at a foundry. The patient was a non-smoker and did not consume alcohol.

PAST MEDICAL HISTORY

The patient's past medical history included an amoebic liver abscess (treated in India). She had no allergies, and apart from painkillers and antiemetics, was on no long-term medication.

SYMPTOMS

This case occurred shortly after I started my new role as a medical registrar at the hospital. The consultant I work for was nearing retirement. One Tuesday evening, he received a request for a domiciliary visit (DV) from a local GP concerning the patient, with limited details provided about her condition. The GP reported that she had been unwell for about two weeks, presenting with vomiting and a headache, alongside a general feeling of malaise. She had no diarrhoea.

EXAMINATION

The GP had visited her twice, diagnosing a viral illness. Four days ago, her son took her to the local hospital's A&E department, where she was discharged with antiemetic tablets, but her condition had not improved. The GP then requested a DV.

During the home visit, the consultant struggled to obtain detailed information due to the language barrier, and the patient was unable to communicate effectively. With limited history and difficulty performing a fundoscopy without dilating the pupils (as the patient could not co-operate due to the language issues), the consultant decided to admit her for further assessment.

At 7:00 pm, the consultant called me from his home, explaining the situation and asked me to give it a try. I headed to the ward just before visiting hours ended, hoping to catch one of her visitors who could speak English.

Upon arrival, found several family members present and managed to speak with someone who communicated in reasonable English. The patient had been experiencing intermittent headaches and vomiting, with no recent travel history outside the UK in the past three years. She had no rash, cough, fever, abdominal pain, shortness of breath, or photophobia. Her vision was fine, and there was no double vision reported.

Observations following examination of the patient were as follows:

- Height: 162 cm
- Weight: 68 kg
- Comfortable and hydrated, no obvious pain or rash, no signs of trauma, and clinically non-anaemic.
- Temperature: 38.2°C
- Pulse: 110 bpm, regular
- Oxygen saturation: 98%
- Blood pressure: 146/78 mmHg
- Fundi: After pupil dilation, no papilledema, haemorrhages, or exudates observed.

- Blood glucose: Normal
- Heart: Normal size, no murmurs, no signs of heart failure.
- Chest: No deformities, normal expansion, vesicular breath sounds, no added sounds.
- Abdomen: No rash, no jaundice, liver palpable 4 cm below costal margins, smooth and non-tender, spleen just palpable, otherwise normal abdominal examination.
- Upper and lower limbs: No abnormalities detected.

What do you think likely diagnosis was?

There was normal response to plantar reflex (flexion of the big toe). The patient exhibited neck stiffness, so a chest X-ray was urgently requested as a quick, simple and cost-effective way to check for signs of tuberculosis (TB).

DIAGNOSIS

Tuberculosis. Later that evening, at 9.30 pm, the Senior House Officer (SHO) contacted me, concerned about the chest X-ray results. Upon reviewing the film, I identified a classic miliary TB pattern.

TREATMENT

The patient was promptly transferred to a specialist TB hospital for further treatment.

Key diagnostic clues included:

- Persistent fever.
- Palpable liver and spleen, a common finding in miliary TB.

- Ongoing vomiting.
- Absence of papilledema, but awareness that choroidal tubercles may be visible in elderly patients.
- Lack of chest signs until late stages, though fine crepitations may develop.

LESSONS LEARNED

- Conducting home examinations can be challenging and may prevent a thorough assessment.
- Poor patient history and language barriers can complicate reaching a diagnosis.
- Always consider common illnesses that may disproportionately affect ethnic minorities.
- Persistent vomiting and headaches should raise suspicion of raised intracranial pressure or meningitis.
- opt for the quickest, simplest, and most cost-effective investigation methods available.
- Public health responsibilities include tracing contacts, especially in infectious diseases like TB.

Case study 36

INTRODUCTION

The seventy-year-old patient, a lifelong resident of west midlands, had spent most of his working life in manual, semi-skilled jobs. He lived alone and had a long history of smoking, averaging ten cigarettes a day for over thirty-five years. Married twice, he had one daughter. His lifestyle was largely unremarkable, and he registered with the GP practice ten years prior to his diagnosis.

SYMPTOMS

Three years before his diagnosis, he presented with an itchy rash in his groin area, which resembled a fungal infection.

TREATMENT (INITIAL)

He was initially prescribed an antifungal cream to apply three times daily. Over the years, he made multiple visits to the practice, seeing different doctors who, each time, treated the condition as a recurring fungal infection. He was even prescribed antibiotics occasionally, in case of bacterial involvement.

SUBSEQUENT TREATMENT

As time passed, the rash worsened and began to spread. During one visit, he reported increased itching and discomfort. The GP, suspecting a fungal infection, prescribed another course of antifungal cream, along with a week's worth of Flucloxacillin. The patient was advised to return for a follow-up after a week, which he did. However, the condition showed no signs of improvement.

At this point, the patient was referred to district nurses for dressing. Upon examination, one of the nurses expressed concern, noting the presence of shiny, non-oozing, red ulceration in the left groin area. She had never seen a lesion quite like it and recommended an immediate referral.

The GP swiftly dictated a referral letter, and the patient was scheduled to see a dermatologist. Unfortunately, due to unforeseen circumstances, the patient missed his dermatology appointment and was discharged from the clinic. After visiting the practice again, requesting a second referral, an urgent appointment was arranged.

Four months later, the patient finally saw the dermatologist and underwent a punch biopsy.

Guess what was the diagnosis?

DIAGNOSIS

The histology results, received by the practice weeks later, revealed a surprising diagnosis: Extramammary Paget disease (EMPD).

Extramammary Paget disease (EMPD) is an extremely rare condition, with only fifty to sixty cases reported annually in England. It is often associated with underlying malignancy and typically affects areas with apocrine glands such as the genital or perianal regions. EMPD often mimics other more common conditions like fungal infections or eczema, making it difficult to diagnose, especially for general practitioners (GPs) who are unlikely to encounter it in their careers.

DIFFERENTIAL DIAGNOSIS

The differential diagnosis for EMPD includes more common conditions such as:

- Eczema
- Psoriasis
- Lichen sclerosis
- Fungal infections

COMPLAINT AND SUBSEQUENT TREATMENT

In this case, despite the patient's eventual diagnosis, a complaint was filed with a solicitor, highlighting the importance of timely referral and accurate diagnosis in unusual cases. The treatment of choice for EMPD is usually surgical, given its association with skin malignancy and the potential involvement of internal organs.

LESSONS LEARNED

This case highlights several important lessons for medical practitioners:

- Consider rare diagnoses: If a condition does not respond to conventional treatment, it is essential to broaden the differential diagnosis and consider less common possibilities, including rare diseases like EMPD.
- Second opinions matter: When in doubt, seeking a second opinion or a specialist referral can prevent delays in diagnosis and treatment.
- Act swiftly on non-responsiveness: If a patient shows no improvement after initial treatment, further investigation is critical. Quick action can prevent missed diagnoses and potential legal complications.

This case of extramammary Paget disease emphasizes the difficulty in diagnosing rare conditions that mimic more common ailments.

It underscores the need for heightened awareness, especially when dealing with non-responsive cases. Although rare, EMPD can have serious implications, particularly if associated with malignancy, making early diagnosis and appropriate treatment crucial.

Case study 37

INTRODUCTION

This sixty-two-year-old Caucasian male had recently retired due to ill-health He had smoked a pack of cigarettes daily since age sixteen and now suffered from chronic obstructive pulmonary disease (COPD). He lived with his wife in a ground floor flat. He consumed alcohol regularly, about two pints daily with increased intake over weekends.

HISTORY

He had a history of upper abdominal pain radiating to the back, accompanied by vomiting with coffee-ground substance. The pain later settled in the right lower abdomen. Apart from the COPD, he also suffered from hypertension, gout, and chronic back pain. His current medication was Tiotropium (18 mcg), beclomethasone inhaler (200 mcg), allopurinol (300 mg), amlodipine (5 mg). He was allergic to Erythromycin.

EXAMINATION

Observations following examination of the patient were as followed:

- General condition: Overweight (100 kg, BMI of 34.6), appeared anxious, mild shortness of breath (RR 18), and a barrel-shaped chest consistent with COPD. He displayed mild cyanosis, congested eyes and warm peripheral extremities.
- Chest findings: Poor chest expansion, hyper-resonance on percussion, and bilateral vesicular breathing with expiratory wheeze and scattered inspiratory crepitations that cleared upon coughing.

- Cardiovascular: Heart rate of 100 bpm, normal heart sounds except for a loud second heart sound in the pulmonary area, no peripheral oedema.
- Abdominal exam: Slight jaundice, right lower quadrant tenderness with rebound tenderness, but no organomegaly or ascites. Faint bowel sounds were noted.
- CNS: Grossly normal.

What was the likely diagnosis?

INITIAL DIAGNOSIS

Acute appendicitis. The acute onset of abdominal pain, which radiated to the right iliac fossa and settled in the right lower abdomen, along with rebound tenderness, led the medical team to initially diagnose the patient with acute appendicitis. A surgical team was consulted, and the patient was scheduled for surgery.

DIFFERENTIAL DIAGNOSIS

- Other possible causes of the acute abdominal presentation include:
- Dissecting aortic aneurysm
- Perforated duodenal ulcer
- Gallbladder disease (cholecystitis or gallstones)
- Hiatal hernia
- Acute pancreatitis
- Kidney stones

What do think the final diagnosis was?

Despite the initial plan for surgery, further investigations prompted the surgeon to reconsider.
The final diagnosis, pancreatitis, was confirmed based on elevated serum amylase levels (2,500 U/L), which strongly suggested pancreatic inflammation. The decision not to proceed with surgery was informed by this key laboratory finding.

Several factors should have pointed towards acute pancreatitis early in the assessment:

- Nature of the pain: The patient's description of upper abdominal pain radiating to the back is a classic feature of pancreatitis.
- Localised tenderness: Although tenderness was more pronounced in the right lower quadrant, this may have been secondary to local peritonitis, caused by fluid leakage from the inflamed pancreas.
- Alcohol consumption: The patient's regular alcohol intake(two pints daily with higher consumption on weekends) was a significant risk factor for pancreatitis. Elevated Gamma-GT levels (126) further supported this.
- Coffee-ground vomiting: While more commonly associated with gastrointestinal bleeding, this symptom can also occur in cases of acute pancreatitis, as part of the systemic inflammatory response.

LESSONS LEARNED

- Non-specific presentations: Acute abdominal pain can present in ways that mimic other conditions, such as appendicitis.

Clinicians should remain open to alternative diagnoses, especially when initial presentations are ambiguous.

- Alcohol history: Patients may underreport their alcohol consumption, potentially leading to diagnostic errors. It is essential to gather a thorough and accurate history.
- Diagnostic work-up: In cases where the clinical picture is unclear, early consideration of acute pancreatitis should be included, especially when key risk factors like alcohol intake and characteristic pain patterns are present.

In conclusion, this case highlights the importance of maintaining a broad differential diagnosis in patients with acute abdominal pain, especially in the presence of risk factors like chronic alcohol consumption.

Case study 38

INTRODUCTION

This sixty-six--year-old male had been registered at the practice for three years. He retired a year previously after twenty-five years as a train driver.

He had never smoked, consumed around 18 pints of alcohol weekly, lived in a council house with his wife and had two grown-up children. He enjoyed regular holidays in and outside the UK, with the last holiday being six months ago.

Following a consultation in 1990, he initially presented with unexplained unsteadiness for three months, without a history of ear problems, hearing loss, ear discharge, sore throat or weight loss. Recently, he experienced intermittent pain in his calf muscles and occasional numbness in his toes, leading to fear of falling and curtailing his daily walks. He followed a balanced diet, takes multivitamins, and consumed plenty of fruit and vegetables.

PAST MEDICAL HISTORY

He was taking atenolol (25mg daily) for well-controlled hypertension and allopurinol for gout. He underwent surgery for a stomach ulcer in 1971. He had no known allergies.

EXAMINATION

Observations following examination of the patient were as follows:

- Physical condition: Well-dressed, mildly anxious but pleasant, and clinically stable.
- Vitals: Weight: 76kg, height: 178cm, BP: 146/78, pulse: 88 bpm (sinus rhythm).

- Cardiovascular and respiratory systems: Normal.
- Abdomen: No abnormal findings (no masses or signs of ascites), liver and spleen non-palpable.
- Central nervous system (CNS): Cranial nerves intact, memory for recent and remote events good. Sensory loss (light touch) over toes. Reflexes normal, with no other neurological abnormalities.

DIAGNOSIS (INITIAL)

What do you think might be the diagnosis at this stage?

TREATMENT (INITIAL)

- Ordered blood tests: FBC, ESR, LFTs, Urea, Electrolytes, Gamma-GT.
- Advised reducing alcohol intake.
- Scheduled a review in one week.

A week late, the flood tests returned normal (LFTs, Calcium, Hb 14g/dL, MCV 86, ESR 10). Gama GT was just above normal. I reassured the patient and advised reassessment in eight weeks after further alcohol reduction.

At the second consultation eight weeks later, there was no improvement; in fact, unsteadiness had worsened, and the patient now avoided going outside due to fear of falling. Reflexes were brisk, and plantar response was extensor.

- Lower limb sensation had deteriorated.
- Repeated blood tests remained normal (Hb 13.5g/dL, MCV 84).

REVISED DIAGNOSIS

Likely upper motor neurone lesion; specific cause uncertain.

I recommended referral to a neurologist and requested. A blood test for syphilis was also requested.

The patient was satisfied with the action plan, and a neurologist appointment was scheduled.

The patient's wife later reported worsening symptoms, including forgetfulness, requiring written notes for reminders, I contacted the neurologist to discuss the case, repeated blood tests and maintained the scheduled appointment

Diagnosis made after additional blood tests requested.

> What blood tests were requested and what was the diagnosis?

DIAGNOSIS

The neurologist identified the problem after additional blood tests: Vitamin B12 deficiency (very low level

The final diagnosis was subacute combined degeneration of the spinal cord.

Initially missed the correct diagnosis. The presence of upper motor neurone signs, sensory loss and eventual memory issues should have alerted me to the possibility of subacute combined degeneration of the spinal cord due to Vitamin B12 deficiency. However, the patient's normal haemoglobin and mean corpuscular volume (MCV) levels misled me.

What do you think the final diagnosis was?

LESSONS LEARNED:

- Normal blood tests don't rule out Vitamin B12 deficiency: Even in cases of severe Vitamin B12 deficiency, the peripheral blood picture can remain normal. This is particularly true when patients are taking over-the-counter multivitamins that contain small amounts of Vitamin B12, which may prevent anaemia but not neurological damage.
- Check Vitamin B12 in cases of neuropathy: In patients presenting with peripheral neuropathy, especially with upper motor neurone signs, it is crucial to check Vitamin B12 and folate levels.
- History of stomach surgery can impair B12 absorption: The patient's surgery for peptic ulcers affected the stomach's intrinsic factor production, leading to impaired Vitamin B12 absorption.
- Early treatment is vital: Although Vitamin B12 injections can correct anaemia, neurological symptoms can persist if treatment is delayed. Early diagnosis and treatment are essential for preventing irreversible damage to the spinal cord and brain.

Case study 39

INTRODUCTION

This sixty-five-year-old retired hotel receptionist from North Wales, lived with her husband in a bungalow.

SYMPTOMS

She had been feeling unwell for three weeks, experiencing weight loss, weakness, poor appetite, and later, shortness of breath. There were no respiratory, gastrointestinal or urinary symptoms.

The patient had been seen by her GP a week prior to hospital admission. The GP noted a low-grade fever (37.6°C) but found no other significant signs, diagnosing her with a possible viral infection and recommending rest, paracetamol, fluids and a balanced diet. A week later, her condition worsened with the development of shortness of breath, prompting referral to the hospital.

PAST MEDICAL HISTORY

Her medical history included a hysterectomy for a prolapsed uterus ten years prior, and she was not on any regular medication.

EXAMINATION

On admission, she was alert and pleasant, without any apparent shortness of breath at ted

Clinical examination revealed a fever of 38°C, a pulse rate of 105 (sinus rhythm), and a blood pressure of 145/82 mmHg. Cardiovascular and respiratory system examinations were unremarkable. No cyanosis, murmurs, or signs of heart failure were detected. The abdomen was soft, with no palpable organomegaly.

Peripheral pulses were palpable, and no oedema was present.

Blood tests requested, results.

- ESR: 70 mm/hr
- Haemoglobin: 10 g/dL (normochromic, normocytic)
- Leucocytosis: 13,000/μL
- Chest X-ray: Normal
- Urine examination: Microscopic haematuria with a few red blood cells

All other tests, including renal function, liver function, and cultures, were initially normal.

> At his stage, what was the probable diagnosis and how would you manage it?

TREATMENT (INITIAL)

no initial evidence of a viral infection, the consultant opted for a conservative approach, administering analgesics and monitoring. Upon re-examination during a ward round, the senior registrar detected a palpable spleen, suggesting a potential systemic condition. Given the presence of microscopic haematuria and leucocytosis, the suspicion of bacterial endocarditis arose.

SUBSEQUENT TREATMENT,

The microbiologist was consulted and advised:

- Collection of three sets of blood cultures from different sites at peak temperatures

- Empirical treatment with double antibiotics (benzylpenicillin and gentamicin).

After three days of antibiotic therapy, the patient's condition improved, and her fever subsided. Blood culture results confirmed the presence of streptococcus viridans, sensitive to the antibiotics administered.

DIAGNOSIS

Bacterial endocarditis, confirmed by positive blood cultures for streptococcus viridans and clinical improvement with appropriate antibiotic therapy.

LESSONS LEARNED

Clinical suspicion and thorough examination:

- The senior registrar's detection of a palpable spleen, combined with the microscopic haematuria and elevated ESR, guided the team towards the correct diagnosis of endocarditis, despite the absence of typical signs such as new heart murmurs.

Key indicators of endocarditis:

- \- Fever and new murmur should raise suspicion of endocarditis until proven otherwise.
- \- Splenomegaly and microscopic haematuria are important clues in the absence of other more obvious symptoms

Blood cultures and empirical treatment:

- Repeated blood cultures from different sites are crucial in diagnosing infective endocarditis, especially in the presence of persistent fever. Early initiation of empirical antibiotics can be lifesaving, even before culture results are available.

Collaboration with specialists:

- Early consultation with both microbiologists and cardiologists ensured timely and appropriate management, highlighting the importance of multidisciplinary teamwork in complex cases.

Mortality and organisms:

- The common causative organism, streptococcus viridians, carries a mortality rate of 6 per cent when appropriately treated. However, more aggressive organisms such as Staphylococcus aureus may result in much higher mortality rates (up to 30 per cent).
- The case underscores the importance of maintaining a high index of suspicion for bacterial endocarditis, even when typical signs are absent. Early diagnostic steps and empirical treatment can greatly reduce the risk of fatal outcomes. Although echocardiograms were not widely available at the time, clinical acumen and the strategic use of blood cultures led to a successful diagnosis and treatment.

Case study 40

INTRODUCTION

This sixty-five-year-old Caucasian female, retired at sixty, with a long-standing history of type 1 diabetes, well-controlled hypertension, and osteoarthritis, joined the practice in 1990 when I was a General Practitioner.

SYMPTOMS

She presented with a ten-day history of left lower abdominal pain, worsened by intermittent constipation, alleviated only partially by over-the-counter painkillers (ibuprofen and paracetamol). She denied urinary symptoms, diarrhoea, vomiting, or blood in her stool, though she reported feeling nauseous.

PAST MEDICAL HISTORY

The patient's medical history included:

- Diabetes mellitus type 1: Long-standing, managed with daily Lantus insulin.
- Hypertension: fifteen-year history, well controlled on amlodipine 5 mg and atenolol 50 mg daily.
- Osteoarthritis: Particularly affecting the knees, with intermittent paracetamol use and a steroid injection in the right knee two years ago.

EXAMINATION

Observations following examination of the patient were as follows:

- Vitals: Pulse 115/min, BP 110/76 mmHg, Temp 38°C, SpO2 98%, RR 20.

- Heart: Normal, no murmurs or abnormal sounds.
- Chest: Clear, no added sounds.
- Abdomen: No masses or jaundice. Tenderness localized to the left lower quadrant with no rebound tenderness.
- Urine examination: No abnormalities detected.

TREATMENT (INITIAL)

Given the persistent left lower abdominal pain, localised tenderness, and raised temperature, I contacted the hospital's surgical team, who accepted her for assessment at the Accident and Emergency (A&E). Her husband transported her to the hospital due to its proximity.

The next day, her husband brought in discharge notes recommending only pain relief. Two days later, she returned to A&E due to worsening pain and was prescribed antibiotics alongside painkillers. However, the pain persisted, and the patient's condition worsened. Her husband requested a home visit, but I decided to facilitate her direct admission to the hospital for further investigation. I emphasised to the on-call surgical team the need for thorough assessment and not to discharge her prematurely.

Unfortunately, three days later, her husband informed the practice that she was in intensive care following emergency abdominal surgery. Tragically, she passed away two days later.

What was the diagnosis?

The patient's final diagnosis was perforated sigmoid diverticulitis.

LESSONS LEARNED

- Hospital discharge concerns: Premature discharges can have severe consequences. GPs must advocate for thorough hospital evaluations, especially when clinical signs suggest a more serious condition.
- Diverticulitis may present subtly but quickly can lead to perforation and peritonitis.

complications

- Standing firm for patient care: When secondary care does not meet the required standard, GPs must remain steadfast in ensuring proper patient admission and follow-up.
- Managing complaints: Following a tragic outcome, grieving relatives may lodge complaints. Ensuring a thorough, professional approach at every stage of care is essential to both patient outcomes and professional security.
- This case is a solemn reminder of the challenges faced in ensuring appropriate patient care across the primary-secondary care divide. Despite multiple visits to the hospital and clear signs of significant pathology - fever, tachycardia and localised abdominal tenderness - the patient was sent home prematurely on several occasions. Diverticulitis, while common, can present variably, making diagnosis challenging. Complications such as perforation can lead to severe outcomes, as seen in this case.

Case study 41

INTRODUCTION

This single thirty-two-year-old Caucasian male had been unemployed for the past twelve months, performing irregular jobs. He lived on the seventh floor of a council flat in Birmingham city centre. He smoked one pack of cigarettes a day and consumed approximately fifteen pints of beer weekly.

In August 1984, having just completed my GP trainee year, I embarked on my first locum position in a single-handed practice situated in Birmingham's city centre. The area was rough, and with limited experience, I faced the challenge of running the practice solo during the GP's overseas annual leave.

SYMPTOMS

Two weeks previously, the patient had complained of painless red lumps on both shins and pain in his right ankle, with some stiffness. The GP at the time reassured him, suggesting a viral infection and recommended paracetamol.

On a second visit to the surgery, it was found that the red lumps were fading, and the right ankle had improved. His left knee was stiff and painful. The patient had difficulty sleeping, and paracetamol was ineffective. The GP prescribed ibuprofen and co-proxamol and advised him to return if needed.

The patient attended the surgery one evening, moving slowly with the aid of two walking sticks. His appearance and strong odour of alcohol and tobacco were notable - perhaps to be expected, given his isolation in his flat. I welcomed him warmly, introducing myself, and he informed me this was his third visit in the last two weeks.

Now under my care, the patient explained that both his right and left ankles and knees were painful, accompanied by lower back pain and morning stiffness lasting approximately forty-five minutes. Additionally, he mentioned a sore red right eye three weeks prior, which had been treated successfully with eye drops at the Birmingham Eye Hospital. He denied any further symptoms.

PAST MEDICAL HISTORY

His past medical history included recurrent tonsillitis in childhood, treated with antibiotics. He had no significant allergies, and his medications included ibuprofen 400mg TDS, co-proxamol two tablets QDS.

EXAMINATION

Observations following examination of the patient were as follows:

- General: Pleasant and co-operative, although visibly struggling to remain still due to back pain. No shortness of breath or signs of anaemia.
- Vitals: Temp 37.5°C, Pulse 100 bpm (regular), BP 125/78 mmHg.
- Eyes; showed no visible abnormalities; throat clear with no ulcers.
- Chest: Normal breath sounds, good expansion bilaterally.
- Abdomen: No lumps, tenderness, or organomegaly.
- Upper limbs: Symmetrical with normal power, no abnormalities detected.
- Lower limbs: Right knee swollen, hot, and tender; both ankles swollen, painful, hot, and tender. No skin discoloration or lumps on the shins.
- Back: Difficult to examine due to excessive pain, no visible rash.

DIFFERENTIAL DIAGNOSIS

- Rheumatoid arthritis: While possible, RA typically affects the joints of the hands and not the distal joints involved here.
- Ankylosing spondylitis: Could be considered, though it usually does not involve the distal joints as in this case.
- Gout: Possible, though gout often presents as monoarthritic rather than polyarthritis, and back pain is not typical.
- Psoriatic arthritis: A consideration, but there are no skin rashes or nail pitting observed.
- Rheumatic fever: Could be, but there's no history of recent tonsillitis and the back is not usually affected.
- Upon further questioning, the patient disclosed that approximately six weeks ago, he attended a sexually transmitted disease (STD) clinic, where he was diagnosed with chlamydia and treated with antibiotics.

What was likely diagnosis?

Given the patient's recent chlamydia infection, migratory arthritis, eye involvement (likely episcleritis), and skin manifestations (suspected erythema nodosum on his shins), the most probable diagnosis is reactive arthritis (Reiter's Disease). His back pain could be attributed to sacroiliac joint involvement, common in reactive arthritis. Contributing factors such as his social isolation, smoking, alcohol consumption and irregular employment are likely to have made him more vulnerable to contracting an STD.

MANAGEMENT

1. Hospital admission:
2. Confirm diagnosis: A hospital stay is necessary to confirm the diagnosis and rule out other causes.
3. Social factors: Due to his poor mobility, unemployment and living situation (isolated and alone), he requires additional care and support.
4. Follow-up: Contact with the hospital a few days later confirmed the diagnosis of reactive arthritis.

LESSONS LEARNED

- Detailed history: A thorough patient history is essential to forming a good diagnostic impression.
- Migratory arthritis: This is a key feature in a few conditions, including rheumatic diseases, hepatitis B and C, Lyme disease, fibromyalgia, and reactive arthritis.
- Social factors: A patient's living conditions, and social circumstances can significantly influence both the diagnosis and the management plan.

Case study 42

INTRODUCTION

This forty-one-year-old man, working as a British Gas engineer, was married with two children, and lived in Sandwell, Black Country. He had a twenty-year history of smoking twenty cigarettes a day but did not drink alcohol.

SYMPTOMS

The patient was referred by his GP after vomiting blood with a coffee ground appearance, accompanied by abdominal distension and dark, loose motions. There was minimal pain, but the abdomen appeared distended like a balloon. The patient noticed these symptoms within the last twenty-four hours. He was immediately referred to the hospital by ambulance under blue lights.

PAST MEDICAL HISTORY

- Back pain: Intermittent, never investigated.
- Mild asthma: Treated with salbutamol inhaler, used as needed.
- Family history: His father died at 51 from a heart attack.

He took diclofenac SR 100 mg once daily and salbutamol inhaler as required. He had no known allergies.

Observations following examination of the patient were as follows:

- General: The patient was alert. He described the vomiting as "effortless" and reported slight abdominal pain. He had been sweating and did not show signs of jaundice.
- Pulse: 115 bpm (irregular).

- BP: 100/60 mmHg.
- Temperature: 38.9°C.
- Abdomen: Distended, with hyper-resonance, but no tenderness. Examination of the liver and spleen was difficult due to the distension.
- Chest: Slight expiratory wheeze noted, otherwise normal.
- PR exam: Runny, black tar-coloured stool (indicative of melaena).
- CNS: No abnormalities noted on gross examination.

TESTS SHOWED

- Haemoglobin (Hb): 8 g/dL (normocytic, normochromic anaemia).
- WBC: 20,000/μL (elevated).
- Platelets: Normal.
- Renal and liver functions: Normal.

How do you manage this case at that time?

- Stabilisation: Cross-matching for blood transfusion and nasogastric suction
- Blood transfusion: Administered along with blood cultures, intravenous broad-spectrum antibiotics, and ECG. The ECG showed atrial fibrillation (AF).
- Imaging: An urgent plain abdominal X-ray was requested to assess for potential bowel obstruction, given the patient's abdominal distension and vomiting. Fluid levels revealed under the diaphragm.

What do you think the final diagnosis was?

The patient was reviewed by the surgical team. After consulting with the attending surgeon, the patient was transferred to the operating theatre. The case was challenging, and during surgery, it was confirmed that the patient had 30 cm of gangrenous ileum, necessitating bowel resection.

DIAGNOSIS

Superior mesenteric artery ischaemia leading to small bowel gangrene.

Lessons learned

- This case exemplifies an acute abdomen with differential diagnoses such as dissecting aneurysm, perforated ulcer, gallbladder disease, appendicitis, bowel volvulus, or intussusception.
- The patient had several risk factors pointing toward an ischaemic cause: a strong smoking history, family history of cardiovascular disease, and the presence of atrial fibrillation.
- The "effortless vomiting" suggested paralytic ileus, with other clues including melaena and abdominal distension.
- The gangrene of the small bowel was likely caused by arterial occlusion, leading to bowel obstruction, peritonitis, and subsequent sepsis. This explains the patient's elevated temperature, black stool, and overall presentation.
- This case underscores the importance of early recognition and prompt surgical intervention in patients presenting with ischaemic bowel disease, particularly in those with significant risk factors for vascular occlusion.

Case study 43

INTRODUCTION

This three-year-old child was born full-term via normal vaginal delivery, and his immunisations were up to date.

PAST MEDICAL HISTORY

His medical history included mild intermittent asthma, atopic eczema and recurrent otitis media, with occasional use of salbutamol inhaler and cetraben moisturiser. There was no history of allergies.

SYMPTOMS

One Friday evening, the parents brought the child to the surgery without an appointment. After discussing with the staff, I agreed to see him. The mother, confident and articulate, explained that her son had been vomiting since early morning, accompanied by central abdominal pain. There was no blood in his stool, but he had vomited several times. She had tried offering boiled water without success, and the vomiting persisted. She observed no skin rash or symptoms of photophobia. By the afternoon, the child developed diarrhoea, which was watery but without noticeable blood. Despite the diarrhoea, the abdominal pain remained, prompting her concern and the decision to visit the practice.

EXAMINATION

The child appeared unsettled but was well-hydrated. His temperature was 37.3°C, pulse 106 bpm, and oxygen saturation 99 per cent. There were no abnormalities in the examination of his throat, heart or ears. His neck showed no stiffness, and his abdomen was soft, with mild discomfort in the central region. Bowel sounds were loud, and his testes were normal.

TREATMENT (INITIAL)

Based on the history and clinical findings, I suspected viral diarrhoea and vomiting. I advised supportive care with fluid intake and prescribed Dioralyte sachets. I reassured the parents that the symptoms should improve within a day or two and emphasised the importance of returning if the child's condition did not improve. The parents were satisfied with this plan.

SUBSEQUENT DEVELOPMENTS

Later that evening, the child's condition worsened, leading the parents to contact out-of-hours (OOH) services. After a brief consultation, OOH dispatched a doctor for a home visit. Following a thorough history and examination, the doctor agreed with the initial assessment of viral diarrhoea and vomiting, noting the absence of recent travel or unusual food consumption. He recommended continued fluid intake and the use of paracetamol.

The next day, the child remained unsettled, and the parents decided to take him to the Accident and Emergency department at the local hospital. Following an examination and full assessment, the hospital doctors were uncertain about the diagnosis and sought a second opinion from the on-call paediatric team. After their evaluation, the paediatric team requested a surgical consultation, and the child was then transferred to the surgical ward for treatment.

What was likely the diagnosis?

DIFFERENTIAL DIAGNOSIS

Diagnosing acute appendicitis in young children can be particularly challenging. Gastroenteritis often presents with similar symptoms of abdominal pain and diarrhoea, and in cases of pelvic appendicitis, localising signs may not be evident in the early stages. It is essential to conduct repeated examinations to assess the development of localising signs, unless the child's condition necessitates immediate intervention.

Additionally, urinary tract infections may mimic appendicitis, as they can cause abdominal pain and frequent urination, potentially secondary to pelvic peritonitis. Microscopic urine analysis is critical in suspected appendicitis cases.

Acute mesenteric adenitis, often linked to upper respiratory tract infections, is another differential diagnosis to consider when abdominal pain is present. Other causes, such as pneumonia or diabetes, may also manifest with abdominal pain but can be distinguished through chest X-rays and blood glucose testing, respectively.

Diagnosis: Acute appendicitis

LESSONS LEARNED

- Diagnosing diarrhoea and vomiting in young children is not always straightforward.
- Acute appendicitis in children is a challenging diagnosis that can be easily confused with other causes of abdominal pain.
- A comprehensive differential diagnosis is vital when evaluating abdominal pain in children.

• When in doubt, it is better to refer the child to the hospital to avoid potential misdiagnosis and unnecessary complications.

Case study 44

The patient was a twenty-eight-year-old male, a non-smoker and non-drinker with a law degree. He had no significant prior medical history and no known allergies or medications.

SYMPTOMS

The patient first noticed a painless thyroid lump three years previously. Initially, he experienced no difficulty swallowing or breathing.

EXAMINATION

The patient was referred to an endocrinologist, who performed a fine needle aspiration biopsy. The results were inconclusive, showing features of Hashimoto's thyroiditis. An ultrasound revealed a thyroid nodule, but it was deemed safe to leave untreated at the time.

SUBSEQUENT DEVELOPMENTS

Several months later, the patient began having trouble swallowing. He consulted a private surgeon who, after examination, referred him to a physician as it was outside his area of expertise. The patient was referred to a local hospital endocrinologist. Despite being marked as an urgent case, his initial appointment was scheduled eight months away. However, arrangements were made for the appointment within two months instead.

Upon seeing the consultant, she advised him that it was not her area and referred him to a surgeon.

TREATMENT

After three months of waiting and further investigations, the surgeon recommended surgery due to the increasing swallowing difficulties. The procedure was successful, and four weeks post-op, the patient was informed that the lump was malignant. However, further screening found no metastasis. Following thorough discussions, the patient opted to remove the remaining thyroid. A second surgery ensued, followed by radioactive iodine treatment, all of which went well.

SUBSEQUENT DEVELOPMENTS

Four weeks after the second surgery, the patient presented to his GP with complaints of burning sensations in his lower limbs, particularly his feet, as well as in his hands. He also noticed occasional skin flickering and increasing fatigue. His condition deteriorated, with daily worsening of the burning sensations and extreme exhaustion.

EXAMINATION

Observations following examination of the patient were as follows:

- General: An intelligent individual with no signs of anaemia, jaundice, or respiratory distress.
- Vitals: Temperature: 37°C, Pulse: 90 bpm (sinus rhythm), Respiratory rate: 18/min, Blood pressure: 124/76 mmHg, Oxygen saturation: 99%.
- Cardiovascular, respiratory, and abdominal examinations were normal.
- Lower limbs: Fasciculations observed in both thighs, with no muscle atrophy. Tendon reflexes and joint movements were

normal, but there was reduced touch and temperature sensation in both feet. Minimal touch sensation reduction was noted in the upper arms.
- Neurological examination: Cranial nerves were intact; Romberg's sign was negative.

SUBSEQUENT TREATMENT

The surgeon corrected the patient's low calcium levels, suspecting it might be contributing to the symptoms, but this provided no relief. The patient was referred to a neurologist, who performed a full examination, including EMG tests, which were all normal. The neurologist also suspected low calcium as a potential cause but found no neuropathy.

At this point, the patient felt his condition was at a standstill. He requested another appointment with the neurologist, having read extensively about his symptoms. He insisted on a skin biopsy, believing it would confirm his self-diagnosed condition, but the neurologist was initially reluctant. Eventually, the neurologist agreed, and the biopsy was sent to Oxford for analysis.

Several weeks later, the hospital called, requesting the patient to meet with the neurologist. The biopsy results confirmed the patient's suspicions.

What was the diagnosis?

SMALL FIBRE SENSORY NEUROPATHY (SFSN)

Small fibre sensory neuropathy is a relatively recently recognised condition; significant advancements have been made in its understanding over the past seven years. It primarily affects the small sensory fibres of the skin, causing symptoms such as burning sensations, pins and needles and severe fatigue.

Common causes include diabetes and pre-diabetes, but in more than half of the cases, the cause remains unknown. Notably, standard tests such as EMG often return normal results, and diagnosis is made only through a skin biopsy, as was the case with this patient. Treatment for SFSN is generally symptomatic and supportive.

This case highlights the pivotal role of patient knowledge in healthcare. The patient's extensive research led to an accurate self-diagnosis, showcasing how technology and access to information empower patients today.

LESSONS LEARNED

- Patient perspectives must be taken seriously – Dismissing patient insights can delay crucial diagnoses.
- Shared care is essential – Collaborative management between specialists and patients can lead to better outcomes.
- Patients are key players in their care – Physicians should view themselves as guides while patients, armed with knowledge, take active roles.
- Seeking help and second opinions is critical – When faced with uncertainty, consulting other professionals can provide clarity.
- Access to knowledge is power – The digital age enables patients to research their conditions and engage more actively in their healthcare decisions.

Case study 45

INTRODUCTION

A twenty-four-year-old single lady recently moved from Kent, in southeast England, to the Black Country in the Midlands, after graduating with a law degree. She joined a solicitor firm and registered with the practice as a new patient. She did not smoke, drank socially, and had no children.

During her new patient check, she mentioned she had been planning to book an appointment for a particular issue.

PAST MEDICAL HISTORY

Her medical history is unremarkable apart from occasional coughs and colds. She was on no regular medication and had no allergies.

SYMPTOMS

She described episodes of blurred vision that had been occurring intermittently for years, with the episodes worsening in the summer. Notably, she experienced no pain, itching, redness, headaches or vomiting. Her GP referred her to a neurologist, who conducted two evaluations. The neurologist found no pathology on examination, nor in the blood tests and CT scan. Given the absence of any significant findings, he advised a watch-and-wait approach, suggesting she return if her symptoms worsened. Dissatisfied, she sought a second opinion.

EXAMINATION

Observations following examination of the patient were as follows:

- Well-dressed, intelligent, and articulate

- Clinically not anaemic, no jaundice or shortness of breath
- Height: 165 cm, Weight: 61 kg, Blood Pressure: 124/76 mmHg
- Cardiovascular and respiratory systems: Normal
- Cranial nerves: Normal except for dilated pupils, which were unresponsive to light or accommodation
- Gait: Normal
- Romberg's sign: Negative

What was the differential diagnosis at that time?

- Drug-induced mydriasis, Common culprits include antihistamines, medications for Parkinson's disease, atropine, and decongestants. However, she was not on any prescribed medications.
- Recreational drug use, substances like amphetamines, cocaine, LSD and ecstasy can cause dilated pupils, but the patient denied using these drugs.
- Benign episodic unilateral mydriasis, a rare condition characterised by episodic pupil dilation and blurred vision without a known cause. Symptoms are transient, like the patient's complaint.
- Adie's pupil (tonic pupil), a rare neurological disorder involving dilated pupils that respond sluggishly to light. It is often associated with absent or poor reflexes. However, no reflex abnormalities were noted in this patient.
- Other causes: Brain injuries or trauma to the eye are rare possibilities, but no history of trauma was mentioned.
- The patient's blurred vision was linked to pupil dilation. However, none of the typical causes appeared to fit her history and examination findings. More details were needed.

What do you think the diagnosis was?

The patient was called back for further investigation. As a previous referral to a neurologist had yielded no answers, she was understandably hesitant to undergo the same process again. Revisiting the history, the patient became irritated by repetitive questions but eventually offered her handbag for inspection. Among her belongings was an antiperspirant product, which she mentioned she used regularly for excessive perspiration.

Upon examining the ingredients, it became clear that the product contained atropine derivatives, which are known to cause systemic side effects, including blurred vision through pupil dilation. The patient acknowledged that she also experienced mild dry eyes and mouth - classic symptoms of an anticholinergic reaction.

DIAGNOSIS

The patient's dilated pupils and blurred vision were attributed to medication-induced anticholinergic side effects from her antiperspirant.

TREATMENT

She was advised to discontinue the use of the product for four weeks, and an alternative antiperspirant (Driclor) was prescribed. Upon her return, she reported that her symptoms had resolved.

This case posed a diagnostic challenge due to the subtlety of the clues. The worsening of symptoms in the summer pointed to increased use of the antiperspirant. The episodic nature of her symptoms further suggested the influence of a topical product rather than a systemic condition. Over-the-counter medications, particularly those applied topically, are often overlooked by patients when recounting their medical history, yet they can cause significant side effects.

LESSONS LEARNED

- A thorough medication history should include over-the-counter products, as they can have systemic effects.
- Seasonal patterns in symptom presentation should be explored, as they may provide important diagnostic clues.
- Topical medications, even when used for benign purposes, can cause serious systemic side effects, particularly when they contain anticholinergic agents.

This case underscores the importance of a detailed and thoughtful approach to history-taking, even when initial investigations fail to yield an answer.

Case study 46

INTRODUCTION

This ten-year-old boy of Polish origin was brought in by his visibly exhausted mother.

His past medical history included mild asthma, managed with salbutamol inhaler on a PRN basis, no known allergies. Family history was significant in that his sister had Crohn's disease.
Symptoms

The child presented with a six-week history of worsening, dull, central abdominal pain. Notably, there was no vomiting, no radiation of the pain, and regular bowel movements without diarrhoea or constipation. His urine was clear, with no blood or pain reported.

TREATMENT (INITIAL)

The child had visited his GP multiple times and the emergency department (A&E) twice, only to be reassured and sent home with painkillers each time. Three days previously, he was admitted to the hospital, given laxatives, and discharged after two nights, with no improvement. Unhappy with the progress, the mother took the boy back to A&E, where he was triaged and referred to an out-of-hours (OOH) service. She expressed deep concern over her son's worsening condition, his inability to sleep, and missed school due to exhaustion and pain.

EXAMINATION

Observations following examination of the patient were as follows:

The child appeared quiet, underweight and slightly pale. His weight was recorded as 25 kg and height 125 cm. Vital signs were within normal limits:

- Pulse: 96 bpm
- Temperature: 37.1°C
- Oxygen saturation: 98%
- Respiratory rate: 20 breaths per minute

No abnormalities were noted in the heart or chest, and no jaundice was present. However, abdominal examination revealed distension and dullness on percussion, with a palpable central abdominal mass measuring approximately 15 cm by 12 cm. No signs of ascites were observed. Other systemic examinations, including CNS and skin, were unremarkable.

What would you do at that time?

TREATMENT OPTIONS

■ Admit the child to the hospital:

Given the recurring nature of the symptoms, multiple prior visits with no improvement, and the mother's legitimate concerns, admission was deemed the most appropriate course. Although the on-call paediatrician initially suggested the child was suffering from constipation, this was not consistent with the clinical picture or past management. Upon further discussion, it was agreed that the child required a more in-depth evaluation for a serious underlying condition, leading to his readmission.

■ Referral back to the GP was considered inappropriate, given the failure of previous treatments, the family's frustration, and the child's worsening condition. This could also have led to a formal complaint from the family, further delaying necessary intervention.

DIFFERENTIAL DIAGNOSIS

- Wilms' tumour (Nephroblastoma): Although Wilms' tumour typically presents with a mass on the side of the abdomen rather than centrally, it remained a consideration. Half of these patients also show signs of elevated temperature and haematuria, neither of which were present in this case.
- Retroperitoneal tumour (adrenal medulla): This diagnosis is difficult to distinguish from Wilms' tumour, especially given the central location of the mass.
- Constipation, despite the treatment with laxatives, the child's condition did not improve, and he had been experiencing regular bowel movements. This effectively ruled out constipation as the primary cause.
- Small bowel B-cell lymphoma: Although rare, this form of lymphoma was a significant consideration due to the presence of a central abdominal mass.
- Hydronephrosis, Given the lack of any prior or recent renal issues, this was considered but less likely.

What do you think the final diagnosis was?

Two days later, a follow-up with the hospital confirmed the diagnosis of small intestine B-cell lymphoma.

LESSONS EARNED

- Discharge does not equal resolution, discharging a patient does not always signify that they have been cleared of any serious underlying conditions. In this case, multiple attendances should have raised more suspicion.

- Take multiple visits seriously, repeated presentations should prompt a thorough re-evaluation, especially when a patient's condition does not improve.
- Consider rare diagnoses, even though small bowel lymphoma is uncommon in children, a dense central mass warrants a high index of suspicion for serious illnesses, including rare ones.
- Advocate for the patient, clinical findings suggest the need for further investigation, it is crucial to stand firm in advocating for admission, even when initial opinions differ.

This case highlights the importance of considering serious underlying conditions in paediatric patients with persistent, unexplained symptoms, even when initial assessments are inconclusive.

Case study 47

INTRODUCTION

The patient was a sixty-year-old Asian widow who recently moved to England. She spoke no English and resided with her daughter's family in suburban Birmingham. The daughter, who acted as the interpreter, mentioned I was the fifth doctor to visit her mother, reflecting her frustration with previous consultations. She had a confrontational attitude, which I understood given the lack of resolution of her mother's symptoms. Despite the earlier visits and treatments, her condition had not improved.

PAST MEDICAL HISTORY

She had had pulmonary tuberculosis which was treated successfully twenty years ago in India. Mild asthma was well controlled with salbutamol. There was no family history of recent illness.

SYMPTOMS

- Onset: eight days prior, marked by persistent vomiting and diffuse headache.
- Symptoms: No fever, rash, sore throat, diarrhoea or limb pain. Mild confusion noticed over the last two days.

EXAMINATION

- General: Appeared exhausted but stable, tolerating light, with a temperature of 37.3°C, pulse 100 bpm, and RR 17.
- Head and neck: Neck stiffness noted, but no other signs of meningism. Clear throat.
- Cardio-respiratory: Mild scattered wheeze on auscultation,

otherwise normal heart and lung sounds.

- Neurological: No motor weakness, normal reflexes, and no cranial nerve deficits. No signs of spasticity or abnormal reflexes.
- Abdomen: Soft, non-tender, no organomegaly.

What was the most likely diagnosis?

- Differential diagnosis
- Subarachnoid haemorrhage (SAH).
- Viral meningitis
- Tuberculous (TB) meningitis
- Meningococcal meningitis
- Stroke
- Transient ischaemic attack (TIA)
- The neck examination revealed neck stiffness, a crucial indicator of potential
- central nervous system involvement.

What do you think the final diagnosis was?

While viral or bacterial meningitis could be considered, the lack of a significant fever or toxic appearance, as well as the absence of a rash, makes these less likely. TB meningitis is a possibility given the patient's history of tuberculosis, but the onset and presentation favour another diagnosis. TIA and stroke are possible but are less likely to account for the full constellation of symptoms, especially in the absence of limb weakness or focal neurological deficits.

Subarachnoid haemorrhage is the most likely diagnosis, based on the following:

- Sudden, persistent headache over several days.
- No fever or rash, ruling out most infections.
- Patient in the right age group for SAH, with additional risk factors, including a history of hypertension or vascular abnormalities.

TREATMENT

Contacted the neurosurgeon on call at the Queen Elizabeth Hospital, Birmingham and explained my suspicion of subarachnoid haemorrhage. The patient was urgently admitted, and a CT scan confirmed SAH. She underwent surgery that night.

Key facts about subarachnoid haemorrhage

- Incidence: 7.9 per 100,000 population.
- Risk factors: Hypertension, smoking, excessive alcohol consumption.
- 85 per cent of cases are due to aneurysms, particularly affecting the circle of Willis (e.g., Berry aneurysms).
- Can present with confusion, seizures, or focal neurological deficits such as hemiparesis.
- Diagnosis: CT scans are 98 per cent accurate in detecting SAH, and this increases to nearly 100 per cent within the first six hours of onset.

LESSONS LEARNED

- Subarachnoid haemorrhage may present atypically: Classical signs like a "thunderclap" headache may not always be evident, particularly in older patients or those with communication barriers.

- Managing frustrated families: Remaining calm and listening to the concerns of family members is crucial, especially when patients have had multiple medical consultations without improvement.
- Act decisively: When faced with ongoing, unexplained symptoms, seek to identify the underlying cause rather than merely treating symptoms.
- Importance of comprehensive examination: Subtle findings such as neck stiffness can direct clinicians toward critical diagnoses.
- This case serves as a reminder of the importance of maintaining vigilance for serious diagnoses even when presentations deviate from the classical textbook descriptions

Case study 48

INTRODUCTION

This seventy-four-year-old male was a retired tailor (he retired eight years earlier); he was a non-smoker and did not drink alcohol. He lived in a second floor flat with his wife. His four children have all left home.

PAST MEDICAL HISTORY

He had hypertension, well managed with amlodipine. His type 2 diabetes was managed with Mixtard 30 (twice daily). He was allergic to penicillin.

SYMPTOMS

- Primary symptom: Central abdominal pain, colicky, lasting around thirty minutes before subsiding. No pain radiation to the back or pelvic area.
- Duration: six months.

EXAMINATION

Observations following examination of the patient were as follows:

- Vitals: Height: 177 cm, weight: 79 kg, BP: 145/78 mmHg, pulse: 96 (regular), temperature: 37.2°C.
- Appetite and weight loss: Patient reported a significant drop in appetite and weight (down to 67 kg).
- No jaundice or palpable lymph nodes
- Abdomen unremarkable
- No thyroid enlargement

Regular bowel movements, no diarrhoea or visible blood in stool, noted occasional constipation, no urinary symptoms

TREATMENT (INITIAL)

Blood tests were ordered by the locum GP. U&E, FBC, LFTs, TFTs, FOB was normal.

Given the patient's progressive weight loss and poor appetite, two options were discussed:

1. Urgent referral
2. Further blood tests to include CRP, ESR, and stool calprotectin

The patient opted for additional blood tests.

Blood test results were as follows:

- CRP: 54 mg/L (elevated)
- ESR: 68 mm/h (elevated)
- Stool Calprotectin: 500 μg/g (elevated)

DIFFERENTIAL DIAGNOSIS, MOST LIKELY.

- Inflammatory bowel disease (IBD), likely Crohn's disease, Colon cancer.

SUBSEQUENT TREATMENT

- Referred for urgent assessment under the two-week wait system.
- Colonoscopy revealed patchy redness in the colon. Biopsies were inconclusive for malignancy, leading to a working diagnosis of Crohn's disease.
- Patient started on high-dose prednisolone with initial improvement (weight gain and symptom relief).

- Relapse occurred during steroid tapering - weight loss, poor appetite and constipation. Laxatives provided minimal relief.
- Given the lack of response to steroids and ongoing constipation, a potential misdiagnosis was suspected.

FURTHER TREATMENT

A second colonoscopy was scheduled, and the patient received a purgative to prepare.

Minimal bowel movement, severe abdominal distension and worsening condition followed.

A CT scan confirmed large bowel obstruction with massive colonic distension.

The patient was taken to theatre for immediate surgical intervention. Upon opening the abdomen, the colon burst due to extreme distension. Fortunately, after surgery and intensive care, the patient survived.

DIAGNOSTIC COMPLEXITY

Misdiagnosis of Crohn's disease without biopsy-confirmed evidence

Over reliance on stool calprotectin as an indicator of IBD without considering other causes (e.g., ca colon).

Delayed recognition of bowel obstruction, which should have been suspected after failure of purgative response.

LESSONS LEARNED

- Stool calprotectin can be elevated in several conditions, including inflammatory, bowel cancer, infective colitis and other causes.

- Confirmed diagnosis through biopsy is essential before treating chronic diseases like Crohn's.
- Steroid treatment failure should prompt reassessment.
- In summary, this case highlights the dangers of premature diagnosis and failure to investigate alternative causes of symptoms. Early identification of obstruction could have prevented a life-threatening situation.

Case study 49

INTRODUCTION

It was 1980, and I was working as a medical registrar in a hospital nestled in the heart of the West Midlands. Our team was on call that weekend, bracing ourselves for the usual rush. The fifty-five-year-old Afro-Caribbean male did not drink alcohol and lived a quiet life with his wife in a semi-detached home. He had worked for Rover for a decade after spending several years as a taxi driver in the Middle East.

Around midday, he was admitted to the medical ward.

SYMPTOMS

His history was troubling: weeks of digestive discomfort that had recently taken a darker turn, quite literally. The man had begun vomiting a black, tarry substance and his stool had assumed the same ominous hue. Abdominal pain gnawed at him, and he was so weak that even the simplest movements left him gasping for air.

EXAMINATION

When I met him, he was polite but visibly worn down, his skin pale beneath its usual tone. His pulse raced at 100 beats per minute, and though his blood pressure held at 140/78, his body was betraying him in quieter ways. His temperature was normal, but when I examined him, the spleen was unmistakably enlarged, palpable five fingers below the costal margin. No glands were swollen, his heart was clear, and his lungs followed suit. On the surface, it didn't appear as though anything sinister was at play, but his worsening anaemia told a different story.

He managed his asthma with salbutamol inhalers as needed and rarely experienced gout flare-ups. Importantly, he had no known allergies, and his lifestyle didn't suggest any obvious risk factors.

But it was his blood results that alarmed us the most. His haemoglobin was a shockingly low 4 g/dL. He was bleeding internally, likely from his stomach or bowels. He had no history of taking aspirin or anti-inflammatory medications, which might have explained the gastrointestinal bleeding. We suspected oesophageal varices, possibly tied to a liver condition. I couldn't ignore the fact that he had lived in the Middle East, where Bilharzia was endemic. It wasn't a stretch to think this parasitic infection might have caused cirrhosis, leading to portal hypertension and the bleeding varices.

TREATMENT

The patient needed immediate stabilisation and a blood transfusion, followed by surgery. I sat down with him, taking a deep breath before explaining what had to happen. "You're bleeding inside, likely from your stomach or intestines," I said. "You need a blood transfusion immediately, followed by an operation. Without the transfusion, we can't stabilise you for surgery."

His answer stunned me. "No blood," he said firmly, citing his religious beliefs. I was taken aback but kept my tone steady. This was life or death, and I had to make him see that. I returned to his bedside four times that day, each time re-explaining the gravity of his situation. Each time, he refused. His beliefs, deeply rooted, seemed unshakable.

What would you do next at that time?

I approached him one last time. My voice was urgent, perhaps more so than before. "This is the last time I'll ask. Without a transfusion, you will almost certainly die. I need your signature now - either to consent or to refuse."

He stared at the form in silence, the weight of his decision pressing down. Time stretched, and then, at last, he nodded. He signed his consent for the transfusion, and soon after, the surgery began.

Thankfully, it was a success. Days later, he walked out of the hospital, alive and on his own two feet - a life saved by the slim margin between conviction and reason.

What was the diagnosis?

OESOPHAGEAL VARICES

This case taught me the vital importance of thorough history-taking and clinical judgement. The enlarged spleen, combined with his history of working in the Middle East, pointed toward Bilharzia, a parasitic infection known to cause liver cirrhosis and portal hypertension, leading to the variceal bleeding he experienced. Without this understanding, the diagnosis might have been missed.

LESSONS LEARNED

- Consent must always be written and documented, particularly in critical situations.

- The patient must fully understand the information and retain it, even in moments of crisis.
- History-taking and clinical findings must always be interpreted in tandem, leading to the correct diagnosis.
- This case illustrates the delicate balance between respecting a patient's beliefs and ensuring they understand the life-or-death stakes at hand.

Case study 50

INTRODUCTION

It was a crisp October weekend in 1980 when I first encountered Mrs T, a sixty-year-old woman, at a hospital. She was a kind-hearted, resilient lady, who, despite the losses and challenges she had faced, radiated warmth and peace. Born and raised in the UK, she had worked for ten years in a foundry, a tough and demanding environment, before moving on to a more nurturing role as a carer for Dos Oak Services, where she spent the remainder of her working life. She retired at sixty-two, and since then lived quietly semi-detached house in the Birmingham suburbs. They were devoted churchgoers, and Mrs T was a regular presence at Sunday services, always humble and content.

She was a non-smoker, didn't consume alcohol, and had no known allergies. She had two daughters - one married and independent, the other tragically lost in a car accident at the age of fifteen. Despite this heartbreaking loss, Mrs. T remained a pillar of quiet strength.

PAST MEDICAL HISTORY

Her medical history was unremarkable, save for her high blood pressure, which had been well managed with amlodipine for the past fifteen years, and some mild pain in her knees, for which she occasionally took simple analgesics.

SYMPTOMS

On this weekend, it was our team's turn to cover the intake, a responsibility that rotated every three weekends among the hospital's three consultant physicians. The patient had been seen first by the houseman in Accident and Emergency, where she presented with worsening shortness of breath. Over the past eight weeks, she had noticed that simple tasks like washing the car or doing housework left her breathless. In the last week, her breathing had worsened to the point where even a flight of stairs became an impossible challenge. She had no cough, wheezing, or phlegm and there was no blood in her sputum. She hadn't noticed any swelling in her ankles, but the shortness of breath was concerning enough for her to visit her GP, who promptly referred her to the hospital.

EXAMINATION

I found her sitting upright, her breathing laboured even at rest. She was cyanosed, her lips and fingers tinged blue, yet she remained calm and pleasant throughout the examination. She stood at 168 cm and weighed 68 kg. Her blood pressure was 142/78, and her pulse was slightly fast at 106 beats per minute, but it was in sinus rhythm. Her jugular venous pressure was not elevated, and her heart sounds were unremarkable. Her respiratory rate was rapid at 28 breaths per minute, with occasional fine crepitations at the lung bases. A neurological exam revealed no abnormalities, and her limbs appeared normal, with no swelling in her ankles.

We quickly initiated investigations:

- Full blood count (FBC): Haemoglobin 8 g/dL, with a mean corpuscular volume (MCV) of 85, indicating normocytic anaemia.
- Urea and electrolytes (U&E): Normal.
- Liver function tests (LFTs): Normal.

- Electrocardiogram (ECG): Showed a rate of 110, but no other abnormalities.
- Chest X-ray (CXR): No obvious abnormalities.
- Arterial blood gases (ABG): Revealed a respiratory acidosis.

Her symptoms and the test results didn't provide a clear diagnosis, and yet there was something unsettling about her case. Her shortness of breath, cyanosis, and respiratory acidosis suggested a respiratory problem, but the normal chest X-ray and absence of signs of heart failure made the picture murky. There was no history of recent travel or immobilisation, yet we couldn't ignore the possibility of a pulmonary embolism.

What would be the next appropriate action at that time?
What was most likely diagnosis?

Consulting the radiologist, we agreed to carry out a ventilation/perfusion (V/Q) scan to assess for possible emboli in her lungs.

DIAGNOSIS, REPEATED SMALL PULMONARY EMBOLI.

The diagnosis was a challenging one to make, but it is not uncommon, especially in elderly, bed-ridden, post-operative or overweight patients. In Mrs T's case, the emboli had likely gone undetected for weeks, her symptoms gradually worsening until she could no longer ignore them. Deep vein thrombosis (DVT) can be difficult to spot, particularly if the clot lies in the pelvic veins, which are not easily visible on routine examination.

LESSONS LEARNED

- When no clear cause can be found for worsening shortness of breath, particularly in vulnerable populations, always consider pulmonary embolism as a possibility.
- Pulmonary emboli often respond well to anticoagulation therapy.
- The absence of visible signs of DVT does not rule out the possibility of emboli.
- A normal chest X-ray does not exclude serious lung pathology.
- While MRI and CT scans are excellent diagnostic tools, a ventilation/perfusion scan remains the first-line investigation for suspected pulmonary emboli.

Mrs T's case was a reminder of the hidden dangers that can lurk beneath seemingly mild symptoms, and how important it is to keep an open mind in diagnosis.

Case study 51

INTRODUCTION

It was a warm summer day in 1984 when I was called to an urgent case during an out-of-hours shift in OOH, the controller's voice carried the weight of concern as they described a man with severe chest pain in a Birmingham suburb. The urgency of the situation left no room for delay, and within minutes, arrived at the address. The house was a large, six-bedroom property, and the patient's wife greeted me anxiously at the door. She led me to a room where her husband sat, his face contorted in pain. He clutched his chest with both hands, his body trembling from the intensity of his discomfort.

As I introduced myself, he looked at me and said with frustration, "Doctor, you're the sixth one they've sent. I've had all sorts of painkillers, but nothing helps." A quick glance at his medication confirmed his claim – he had been prescribed multiple NSAIDs and pain relief without any effect.

SYMPTOMS

The patient's history revealed seven days of persistent chest pain. It was non-radiating, with no associated symptoms like cough, sweating or indigestion. He denied any recent illnesses, injuries or rashes. He was Afro-Caribbean, making subtle physical signs like rashes potentially harder to detect. He was otherwise healthy, working as a solicitor, with no history of smoking or significant alcohol consumption.

EXAMINATION

I immediately began my examination, starting with his vital signs. His blood pressure was 148/90, his pulse was steady at 90 beats per minute, and his temperature was slightly elevated at 37.6°C. His lungs were clear, and there were no abnormal breathing sounds. Listened to his heart carefully, and it was here that I detected something unusual – a subtle rub that hinted at a possible underlying cause for his pain.

TREATMENT

Trusting my instincts, administered a dose of pethidine to provide immediate pain relief and called for an urgent ambulance. While waiting, I contacted the hospital's medical on-call team and emphasised the need for a thorough investigation. I carefully documented my findings and prepared a detailed referral letter. I advised the patient not to read the letter before handing it to the receiving physician, emphasising the importance of a full clinical assessment.

Two years later, while working another out-of-hours shift, was called to the same address, recognised it immediately, even before hearing the patient's name. When he greeted me, hardly recognised him – he had gained significant weight and looked like a different person.

> What was the unusual sound detected on chest examination on my first visit?
> What do you think happened to the patient in the last two years, particularly finding him a lot of weight?

DIAGNOSIS.

The patient's condition had been identified as pericarditis, but further investigation revealed that the underlying cause was systemic lupus erythematosus (SLE). The unusual sound was pericardial rub

TREATMENT

Steroids were used to manage his condition, and these had contributed to his significant weight gain.

This case highlights the importance of listening to patients and trusting clinical instincts. His repeated calls for help were not signs of exaggeration but cries for a diagnosis that had eluded others.

LESSONS LEARNED

- Persistent symptoms warrant deeper investigation: Repeated presentations are often indicators of an undiagnosed condition rather than patient overreaction.
- Act swiftly and decisively: Relieving pain and arranging urgent transport ensured the patient received timely care.
- Thorough examination can be lifesaving: A simple auscultation revealed the clue to his diagnosis.
- Holistic care involves follow-up: Knowing the long-term outcome of cases strengthens professional growth and patient trust.

This case serve as reminders that beneath every symptom lies a story waiting to be uncovered. Our role as clinicians is to listen, investigate and act with compassion and precision to ensure the best possible outcomes for our patients.

Case study 52

INTRODUCTION

In the summer of 1980, while working at one of the hospitals in the West Midlands, I encountered a challenging case involving a twenty-three-year-old woman. She was twenty-four weeks pregnant with her first child and had a history of type 1 diabetes. Apart from her diabetes, she had led a healthy life and was under regular antenatal care. She had no known allergies, was of average height and weight, and was solely dependent on insulin to manage her condition.

SYMPTOMS

She had been admitted to the medical ward following a hypoglycaemic episode, having felt unwell two hours after her last dose of short-acting insulin, which she took four times daily.

EXAMINATION AND TREATMENT

Upon admission, an intravenous cannula was inserted, and a glucose drip was started. Despite this, her condition did not improve significantly. Her initial blood glucose reading was 3.5 mmol/L, and she exhibited extreme agitation and physical resistance, requiring three nurses to manage her.

SUBSEQUENT DEVELOPMENTS

Recognising the urgency of the situation, the senior house officer administered 50 ml of 50% glucose intravenously. After waiting fifteen minutes with minimal improvement, her blood glucose was rechecked and found to be 5.4 mmol/L. A second ampoule of glucose was given, considering that excessive glucose in such cases does not typically cause harm. Five minutes later, her condition improved markedly. She became calm and, soon after, was entirely herself again. A meal was provided to help sustain her blood glucose levels, and her insulin regimen was reviewed and adjusted in consultation with the obstetric department.

LESSONS LEARNED.

- First, it underscored the importance of ruling out other potential causes of such symptoms, including brain tumours or encephalitis, to avoid misdiagnosis.
- Second, learned how severe glucose deprivation can affect the brain, reinforcing the urgency of timely intervention.
- Finally, came to understand that even when blood glucose levels appear within a normal range, individual responses can vary. It is crucial to assess symptoms holistically and tailor treatment to the patient's unique needs.

This experience profoundly shaped my approach to managing complex medical situations, especially in vulnerable populations such as pregnant women. It reinforced the importance of swift decision-making, thorough assessment, and multidisciplinary collaboration.

Case study 53

INTRODUCTION

One early evening in Birmingham City Centre, a twenty-seven -year-old man walked into the out-of-hours (OOH) service with his partner. He appeared anxious but otherwise looked well.

PAST MEDICAL HISTORY

He shared a brief medical history, including an appendectomy five years earlier, chronic otitis media, and mild asthma that only required occasional use of a salbutamol inhaler. He was not on any regular medications and denied using illegal drugs.

SYMPTOMS

His story was straightforward: for the past three days, he had noticed redness on his right buttock, which was now painful. He mentioned feeling feverish and unwell, though he had not experienced any vomiting, diarrhoea or breathing difficulties.

EXAMINATION

The clinical examination seemed to match his story. His vital signs were reassuring: a temperature of 37.6°C, a pulse of 100 beats per minute, and blood pressure within normal limits at 135/82 mmHg. His lungs were clear, his heart sounded normal, and there were no signs of lymph node enlargement or organ swelling. The redness on his right buttock measured about 5 cm by 4 cm, soft to touch with no signs of fluid collection, crusting or oozing. Everything pointed to cellulitis - a relatively common infection - and an appropriate course of oral antibiotics was discussed.

TREATMENT

However, the consultation took an unexpected turn when the patient and his partner began pressing for an injection to relieve his discomfort. Despite explaining that an injection was unnecessary, they insisted. Weighing the situation, I decided to administer a single dose of intramuscular diclofenac for pain relief in his left buttock, ensuring the area was cleaned with a spirit-soaked towel. A prescription for flucloxacillin and advice to take paracetamol as needed completed the visit. He left seemingly reassured, with little hint of what was to come.

SUBSEQUENT DEVELOPMENTS

Two months later, a letter arrived - a complaint that unfolded the story further. The man alleged that the injection I had given him caused his condition to deteriorate. He claimed the injection site had been cleaned improperly, using what he described as a "kitchen towel". According to the letter, two days after our consultation, he presented to the hospital's Accident and Emergency department as his symptoms had worsened. He was sent home with a different antibiotic but returned two days later, now in critical condition.

What do you think why he was in critical condition and possible diagnosis?

DIAGNOSIS AND SUBSEQUENT TREATMENT

The patient were diagnosed with necrotising fasciitis. He underwent extensive surgery to remove infected muscle from his right buttock and thigh. He narrowly survived, spending three weeks in the hospital, and faced a long recovery.

The complaint accused me of negligence, focusing on the injection and alleged improper cleaning technique. With the support of the Medical Defence Union (MDU), I reviewed the case thoroughly. My records showed that I had followed clinical guidelines for cellulitis management, and there was no evidence that the injection contributed to the catastrophic progression of his condition. Necrotising fasciitis is a rare and aggressive infection, often challenging to distinguish from cellulitis in its early stages. The case was closed with no further action, but the experience left lingering questions about what could have been done differently.
Lessons learned

REFLECTING ON THE CASE,

- I recognised areas for growth and improvement.
- Record-keeping stood out as a crucial lesson. While my notes were sufficient to support my clinical decisions, more detailed documentation, particularly regarding the injection process and the rationale behind it, might have strengthened my defence. The allegation about the "kitchen towel" highlighted how even minor oversights in communication or documentation can become focal points in complaints.
- Another lesson lay in the tension between patient-centred care and clinical judgement. While the decision to administer the injection was made to address the patient's immediate concerns, I wondered if a firmer stance on avoiding unnecessary interventions might have been wiser.
- In hindsight, earlier recognition of red flags, such as the severity of the patient's pain or the potential for rapid

progression, could have prompted a referral to secondary care, though this is easier to see with the clarity of retrospect.

The complaint process itself was a reminder of the emotional and professional challenges of practising medicine. Complaints can feel personal, but they also provide an opportunity for reflection and growth. This case reinforced the importance of maintaining professionalism, empathy and an unwavering commitment to evidence-based care, even under pressure.

Necrotising fasciitis is a devastating condition, often striking without warning and progressing rapidly. This case served as a stark reminder of its diagnostic challenges. It also underscored the importance of vigilance, thoroughness and humility in medical practice. For me, it became a story not just of a rare diagnosis but of the balance every clinician must strike between knowledge, judgement and the human elements of care.

Case study 54

INTRODUCTION AND SYMPTOMS

A twenty-two-year-old woman, recently a mother, presented with persistent lower back pain following the birth of her baby boy, a healthy 3.5-kilogram child. Her labour had included an intramuscular injection of pethidine in her right buttock, administered to manage her pain. A day later, she was discharged home, seemingly well. However, just a few hours after the injection, she began to feel discomfort in her lower back.

TREATMENT (INITIAL)

Initially mild, the pain was non-radiating and manageable with paracetamol and ibuprofen. As the days turned into weeks, however, the pain persisted and became resistant to these medications. Convinced that the injection was the source of her discomfort, she sought help from a local physician. He conducted a thorough examination, found no signs of infection or swelling at the injection site, and reassured her that the pain would likely settle with stronger painkillers. Reassured, she returned home.

SUBSEQUENT DEVELOPMENTS

Her partner, concerned about her ongoing distress, contacted me from overseas. After reviewing her history, I noted the absence of pain radiation, trauma, sensory changes or red flag symptoms like bowel or bladder dysfunction. I strongly suggested she obtain an MRI scan and send me the results. However, nine weeks passed without any follow-up, and I assumed her condition had improved.

By chance, I found myself visiting her area and decided to

stop by her home. To my surprise, her situation had deteriorated significantly. She now struggled to sleep and could barely walk due to the escalating pain. Still, both she and her partner remained adamant that the injection was to blame and believed an MRI would be futile.

What would be your action plan at this point?

I conducted another physical examination and found no motor weakness, sensory loss or reflex abnormalities. Blood tests, including FBC, ESR, and liver and renal function tests, were all normal. At this point, I emphasised that the pain was unrelated to the injection and insisted she undergo an MRI to identify the underlying cause.

DIFFERENTIAL DIAGNOSIS

- Sacral strain after labour: The physical stress of labour can strain the sacral and lumbar regions, though this typically resolves with rest and time.
- Postpartum pelvic girdle pain: Hormonal changes during pregnancy lead to ligament laxity and pelvic instability. This usually presents bilaterally, making it less likely in this case.
- Injection-related pain: Localised gluteal pain from inflammation or fatty necrosis at the injection site was possible but unlikely due to the absence of local signs.
- Disc pathology: A herniated disc or discitis could result from the mechanical strain of labour, presenting as persistent and worsening back pain.

What do you expect the finding in the MRI if any?

DIAGNOSIS

The MRI confirmed a disc herniation, a condition likely precipitated by the intense physical strain of labour. This diagnosis validated the need for thorough and timely imaging and redirected treatment toward managing the herniation effectively.

In cases like this, the MRI can show:

- Disc herniation: A protruding disc compressing nearby nerves, as was confirmed here.
- Disc degenerative changes: Early wear and tear exacerbated by the stress of labour.
- Sacral oedema: Inflammation or swelling in the sacral area due to labour-related stress.

LESSONS LEARNED

This case was a stark reminder that assumptions, whether made by patients or physicians, can delay crucial diagnoses. While the patient was fixated on the injection as the source of her pain, the real culprit lay elsewhere, requiring a broader perspective and the persistence to uncover it.

For clinicians, it underscored the importance of balancing empathy with assertiveness, particularly when guiding patients toward necessary investigations. Persistent back pain postpartum should never be dismissed, as labour places tremendous stress on the spine. By pursuing a systematic approach, we can uncover the underlying cause and provide relief to patients like this young mother, who simply wanted to enjoy her new role without the shadow of unrelenting pain.

Case study 55

INTRODUCTION

The patient, M.D., was registered at our practice in the early 2000s while I was working as a general practitioner. She was a thirty-five-year-old woman, highly dedicated to her profession, managing a nursing home for several years. Known for her cheerful and positive demeanour, she rarely visited the practice and had no significant physical or mental health issues. She was the mother of a seven-year-old daughter.

DEVELOPMENTS

However, her life took an unexpected turn when she discovered her husband's infidelity. Initially, she experienced denial and disbelief. Once she fully grasped the situation, she became overwhelmed with confusion and distress, leading to a temporary loss of capacity. In this state, she ingested approximately sixty tablets of 500 mg paracetamol - an overdose with potentially fatal consequences.

Her husband, recognising the severity of the situation, promptly called emergency services. Upon arrival, the ambulance crew was acutely aware of the six-hour critical treatment window for paracetamol toxicity. However, the patient refused to be transported to the hospital. Demonstrating professionalism and sound judgement, the ambulance team remained outside her residence and contacted our practice for further guidance.

It was a summer day, and I happened to be the on-call doctor. Fortunately, her residence was close to the practice, allowing me to arrive within minutes. The ambulance crew was still on site when I reached the scene.

On arrival, I found M.D. in a highly agitated and emotionally distressed state, refusing any hospital attendance or treatment. She was in shock, struggling to process the situation and unable to comprehend the life-threatening risk she faced.

With no history of major illnesses, aside from mild asthma, for which she occasionally used a salbutamol inhaler, M.D. was generally in good health. She was neither a smoker nor a habitual drinker and had no known allergies. However, at this critical juncture, she exhibited a temporary loss of capacity, necessitating urgent intervention within the crucial six-hour timeframe.

At this point what would be your action plan?

Recognising the gravity of the situation, I took a step back for a moment to assess the best approach. I attempted to reason with her, emphasising the severity of her condition and encouraging her to make an informed decision. Despite these efforts, she remained highly agitated and increasingly resistant, showing signs of escalating aggression.

Understanding the time-sensitive nature of the case, I made the difficult decision to involve law enforcement. The police were contacted to provide support in case enforced medical intervention became necessary. Simultaneously, I reached out to the crisis intervention team for immediate psychological support.

Within minutes, two police cars arrived. After thorough discussions, and with persistent efforts from the crisis team, M.D. reluctantly agreed to be transported to the hospital. Their involvement proved instrumental in facilitating her compliance.

So, when is it justifiable to override patient autonomy? The

Mental Capacity Act 2005 provides guidance on such cases. A patient is deemed to lack capacity if they are unable to understand, retain or weigh the necessary information to make an informed decision. In this case, M.D. exhibited a clear loss of capacity, justifying intervention in her best interests to prevent harm.

LESSONS LEARNED

- Acting swiftly in cases of temporary loss of capacity. Healthcare professionals must respond decisively when a patient lacks capacity, ensuring timely intervention.
- The importance of a multidisciplinary team. A collaborative approach involving ambulance services, crisis teams, law enforcement, and hospital staff leads to better patient outcomes.
- Effective communication and empathy Clear, compassionate communication plays a crucial role in crisis management.
- Comprehensive record-keeping Detailed documentation ensures transparency, accountability, and a clear decision-making trail.
- Upholding duty of care. Ensuring that patient welfare remains the primary ongoing professional development.
- Reflecting on this case reinforces my commitment to continuously enhancing my crisis management skills.
- Building and maintaining patient trust. Establishing a strong rapport with patients is fundamental to effective medical care.

This case presents a critical reflection on the management of an acute overdose, addressing both the ethical and intellectual challenges involved. It prompts an important question: how do we balance respect for patient autonomy with the necessity for medical intervention in a life-threatening situation where capacity is lost?

It reaffirmed my dedication to professional growth and reinforced the importance of teamwork, communication, and ethical responsibility in patient's care.

Case study 56

In January, a 20-year-old Afro-Caribbean female presented to the surgery accompanied by her concerned mother. She was holding onto her mother's arm to prevent falling due to an unsteady gait. I stood up and assisted her to sit down safely.
Her mother began explaining the history.

Two weeks prior, the patient developed flu-like symptoms. She self-medicated at home, but her condition did not improve. Nine days later, her mother took her to the local Accident & Emergency (A&E) department.

After assessment, A&E staff diagnosed a probable viral illness, prescribed a course of amoxicillin, and discharged her.

Mother observed increasing difficulty with walking, frequent falls, persistent fever, and a severe cough. Concerned, she returned to the hospital that night and waited for three hours. Despite reporting her daughter's worsening unsteadiness, the hospital reiterated it was likely a viral illness and advised to continue the antibiotics.

Unsatisfied, the mother contacted our practice and booked an appointment for the evening surgery.

HISTORY

On review, the patient reported that her symptoms began with a sore throat and runny nose. She denied haemoptysis, wheezing, or shortness of breath. Her main concern was feeling extremely fatigued, experiencing body aches, and being very unsteady on her feet. She denied vomiting and had not travelled outside the UK in the last two years.

PAST MEDICAL HISTORY:

- Atopic eczema and mild childhood asthma – both resolved, no ongoing treatment.

ALLERGIES:

- No known drug allergies.

CURRENT MEDICATION:

- No regular medication. Took paracetamol. Not on contraception.

SOCIAL HISTORY:

- Lives with her mother in a first-floor flat.

EXAMINATION FINDINGS:

- Appearance: Anxious and low in mood.
- No signs of respiratory distress, bruising, or visible rash (noting it may be harder to detect on darker skin).
- No cyanosis or visible anaemia.
- **Vitals:**
    - Pulse: 98 bpm, regular
    - Temperature: 37.9°C
    - Oxygen saturation: 98%
    - Blood pressure: 125/75 (sitting), 130/82 (lying down)
- **Respiratory Exam:**
    - Trachea central
    - Normal chest expansion
    - Clear breath sounds bilaterally, no added sounds
- **Cardiovascular Exam:**
    - Normal heart size and sounds, no murmurs or pericardial rub
- **ENT & Neck:**
    - Throat clear
    - Ears: minimal wax, drums visible, no signs of infection

- Neck: soft, no stiffness, lymphadenopathy, or palpable lumps

- **Abdominal Exam:**
  - Soft, non-tender, no masses. Not pregnant (last menstrual period 3 weeks prior).
- **Musculoskeletal:**
  - No swelling, joint deformities, or tenderness
  - Spine: no tenderness
- **Neurological:**
  - Cranial nerves: intact
  - Lower limb reflexes were later found to be absent

CLINICAL

1. What would you do next?

I believed the patient required urgent hospital admission. I contacted the on-call medical registrar, who agreed to assess her in the A&E department. I provided a referral letter emphasizing the clinical concerns and the importance of not discharging her prematurely.

2. Do you need any further information to reach a diagnosis?

Yes, a more thorough neurological assessment and possibly lumbar puncture, nerve conduction studies, and CSF analysis would be essential.

3. What do you think might be wrong with the patient?

The history of progressive unsteadiness, recent viral illness, and absence of lower limb reflexes raised strong suspicion of **Guillain-**

FOLLOW-UP

I contacted the medical registrar the next morning. Surprisingly, he reported that he had not seen the patient and was unaware of her whereabouts, as A&E had not contacted him. Upon speaking to the A&E department, I learned that their team had assessed her and discharged her without informing the medical team.

The patient did not return to our practice, and we had no current phone number to follow up. A letter was sent, but no response was received. We were left with no option but to wait for her to re-engage with the service.

Six weeks later, our practice was contacted by a university hospital requesting additional medical information. It was revealed that the patient had been taken privately to a neurologist, who promptly referred her to the Queen Elizabeth Hospital. She required ventilation and narrowly survived.

DIAGNOSIS

Guillain-Barré Syndrome (GBS) – confirmed by absent lower limb reflexes, subsequent neurological deterioration, nerve conduction studies and electromyography

LESSONS LEARNED

- There was a clear failure in clinical and management procedures at the A&E department.
- It is essential to closely follow up with patients presenting with potentially serious conditions, especially when symptoms worsen despite initial treatment.
- Clear communication and escalation between primary care, A&E, and specialist services are critical to avoid missed

diagnoses and delays in care.

- Vigilance is required when a patient reports progressive neurological symptoms such as unsteadiness or weakness following viral illness.